Am I Allowed?

Am I Allowed:

what every woman should know **<u>before</u>** she gives birth

4th Edition

Beverley Ann Lawrence Beech

Birth Practice and Politics Forum

Am I Allowed

Fourth edition published 2021 by Birth Practice and Politics Forum
Edinburgh

©Beverley Ann Lawrence Beech

Beverley Ann Lawrence Beech has asserted her moral right to be named as the author of this work in accordance with the Copyright, Designs and Patents Act 1988.

ISBN-10: 1-9160606-0-9
ISBN-13: 978-1-9160606-0-9
Also available as an e-book

Cover design by Nikki Chhokar

All rights reserved. No part of this book may be reproduced or transmitted in any form by any means for any commercial or non-commercial use without the prior written permission of the author. This book is sold subject to the condition that it shall not, by way of trade and otherwise, be lent, resold, hired out or otherwise circulated without the publisher's prior consent in any form, or binding, or cover other than that in which it is published and without a similar condition being imposed upon the subsequent purchaser.

This book offers general information for interest only and does not constitute or replace individualised professional midwifery or medical care and advice. Whilst every effort has been made to ensure the accuracy and currency of the information herein, the author accepts no liability or responsibility for any loss or damage caused, or thought to be caused, by making decisions based upon the information in this book and recommends that you use it in conjunction with other trusted sources of information.

About the author

Beverley Ann Lawrence Beech is an author, freelance writer, researcher, campaigner, mother of two sons, and has three grandchildren. She has campaigned to improve maternity care since the birth of her second son in 1976.

She was Honorary Chair of the Association for Improvements in the Maternity Services from 1977 to 2017. For six years she was lay adviser to the National Perinatal Epidemiology Unit at Oxford; for seven years a member of the Professional Conduct Committee of the Nursing and Midwifery Council (NMC); and for 5 years a member of the Midwifery Committee of the NMC. She was also a lay member of the Royal College of Obstetricians and Gynaecologists Maternity Forum; a founder member of CERES (Consumers for Ethics in Research); a London Fellow of the Royal Society of Medicine; and a founder member of ENCA (European Network of Childbirth Associations). She is currently a member of the Birth Practice and Politics Forum www.birthpracticeandpolitics.org. She lectures, both nationally and internationally, on women's rights in maternity care and the medicalisation of birth. In her free time she sails, and is President of the London Corinthian Sailing Club.

In 2017, at the Women's Voices Conference at the Royal College of Obstetricians and Gynaecologists, Beverley was presented with an award for her *'Commitment to Improving Maternity Services and Complete Dedication to Women.'*

The Birth Practice and Politics Forum
The Birth Practice and Politics Forum comprises a group of midwives, researchers and birth activists who believe that maternity care in the UK and Ireland is in crisis. Most women are not being nurtured during pregnancy and birth in ways that support their abilities to give birth physiologically. Midwives are not being supported to use their knowledge and skills to provide the kind of care which research

repeatedly shows improves physical, emotional and psychological outcomes for mothers and babies. Maternity services are increasingly influenced by ideological and financial considerations rather than by what is best for women, babies, families and health practitioners.

The Forum regularly posts blogs. You can receive our posts as they are published by putting your email address into the subscribe bar at www.birthpracticeandpolitics.org.uk.

Acknowledgments

In 1983, after many years advising parents, and professionals, of parents' rights, I wrote a booklet *Denial of Parents' Rights in Maternity Care* which, in 1987, developed into *Who's Having Your Baby?* It was the first book to clarify parents' rights in maternity care, and in due course I was encouraged to update it and produced what became *Am I Allowed?*

My late father, Charles Leslie Lawrence MBE, enabled me to do so by financing a lap-top computer, without which *Am I Allowed?* would not have happened. My late husband, Gavin Robertson, encouraged and supported me to update a third edition, and this is now the fourth edition, which is intended to address and reflect the considerable changes that are taking place in the maternity services.

I am also very grateful for the huge amount of invaluable support, comments and assistance I have had from Sarah Davies, Mavis Kirkham, Jean Robinson, Helen Shallow, Vicki Williams and, especially, from Gill Boden, Nadine Edwards and Sara Wickham for their above and beyond suggestions. Much gratitude also goes to the multitude of women who have told me their stories and encouraged me to find out more, to help them make their own decisions about the kind of care they want. My thanks also to Nikki Chhokar who designed the lovely cover.

This book is dedicated to my friend, midwife, and fellow sailor, the late Mary Cronk MBE (1932-2018). Mary was a wonderful, highly skilled midwife, who was a source of support, information and advice. She supported a woman's right to decide what care was appropriate for her, increased my knowledge of clinical issues, and motivated my desire to help women achieve the kind of birth that was best for them.

Contents

Foreword	i
My experience of maternity care	v
Acronyms used in this book	viii
Introduction	1

Chapter 1	The Complexities of Choice	5
	A little bit of history	5
	Choice and decision making	7
	Guidelines	9
	Your decisions and the responsibilities of the midwife	10
	Birth Plans	11

Chapter 2	Planning Ahead: Who Will Attend You?	13
	Considering your options	13
	The implications of Covid-19	14
	Choosing your birth supporters	14
	Midwives	16
	Consultant midwives	17
	Private/independent midwifery care	17
	Private Midwives	18
	Independent midwives	18
	General Practitioner (GP) services	19
	Obstetric services	19
	Health visitor services	20
	Medical and/or midwifery student services	20
	Second opinion	20

	Changing your service provider	21
	Changing your midwife	21
	Changing your obstetrician	22
	Changing your health visitor	22
	A professional's right of access to your home	23

Chapter 3	Planning Ahead: The Kind of Birth You Want	25
	A normal birth	25
	"Overdue" babies	27
	Medically advised caesarean surgery	29
	Reasons for planning caesarean surgery	31
	Vaginal Birth after Caesarean (VBAC)	32
	Consent forms	33
	A water birth	34
	Heated water pools	36
	Freebirthing	37

Chapter 4	Planning Ahead: Place of Birth	39
	Where you give birth is your decision	39
	Options for place of birth	40
	Informed choice for a hospital birth	40
	Do I have to decide early on where to give birth?	41
	Outcomes for different places of birth	41
	Out of hospital settings	43
	Home births	44
	Your right to a home birth	44
	Home birth provision	45
	Inappropriate reasons for suggesting that a home birth is not possible	46
	What if I am told there are not enough midwives?	47
	What to do if your midwife is not supportive	48

	How to secure midwifery services when you are in labour at home	49
	Two midwives attending a home birth	49
	Home birth after a caesarean (HBAC)	51
	Postnatal examination of the baby at home	51
	Free-standing Midwifery Unit (FMU)/ Birth Centres	51
	Alongside Midwifery Unit (AMU)	53
	Consultant Units (OUs)	53
Chapter 5	Antenatal Services	57
	Confirming your pregnancy	57
	Organising antenatal care	57
	Frequency of antenatal appointments	58
	Choosing antenatal classes	59
Chapter 6	Screening and Diagnostic Tests	61
	Body Mass Index (BMI)	63
	Blood pressure (BP)	64
	Urine testing	64
	Blood tests	65
	Screening tests for rare conditions	66
	Diagnostic tests	66
	Domestic abuse	67
	Ultrasound	67
	Doppler devices	69
	Keepsake videos	69
	Ultrasound for low-lying placenta	69
	Ultrasound for estimating baby's weight	70
	Research studies	71
	Human brain development	71
	Accepting or declining ultrasound examinations	72

Chapter 7	Decision Making in Late Pregnancy, Labour and Birth	73
	Stretch and sweep	73
	Induction of labour	74
	Hospital admission criteria	75
	Amniotomy – Breaking the waters or Artificial Rupture of Membranes (ARM)	76
	Electronic Fetal Heart Monitoring (EFM)	77
	Electronic Fetal Heart Monitoring (EFM) during labour	77
	Vaginal examinations (VEs)	78
	Birth positions	80
	Eating and drinking	81
	Time limits	81
	Pain relief	82
	Epidural anaesthesia	83
	Meconium staining	84
	When a baby needs resuscitation	85
	Birthing your placenta	85
	Clamping and cutting the baby's umbilical cord	86
	Cord blood collection	87
	Lotus birth	89
	Who owns your placenta?	89
	Premature, low birth weight or ill babies	90
	When a baby needs neonatal care	90
Chapter 8	After the Birth	93
	Checking your baby	94
	Feeding your baby	95
	Breastfeeding	96
	Vitamin K	98

	The NHS Newborn Blood Spot (NBS) Screening formerly known as the Guthrie Test	99
	When there is a disagreement	99
	If the baby needs to be transferred to a different hospital	100
	When to leave hospital	101
	Leaving hospital against medical advice	101
	A woman's right to stay in hospital	102
	Notifying and registering your baby's birth	102
	Birth notification	102
	Birth registration	103
Chapter 9	Making A Complaint About Your Care	105
	Obtaining a copy of your case notes	105
	Obtaining a copy of your social services notes	107
	False or incorrect information	108
	Your right to obtain statistical information	108
	Your future options	109
	When you are out of time for an investigation of your complaint	110
	Resolving your complaint	111
	Taking legal action	111
	Private care	112
	Transforming maternity care	112
	A serious patient safety incident (SPSI)	113
Chapter 10	When Things Don't Go to Plan: Difficult Outcomes	115
	Extremely premature babies	115
	Miscarriage	116
	Stillbirth and neonatal death	118
	A doctor's duty of care following the death of a baby at birth	119

Post-mortem (autopsy) examination	119
A Coroner's inquiry	120
Dealing with grief	120
Court ordered caesareans	121
Postnatal depression (PND) and	
Post Traumatic Stress Disorder (PTSD)	122
Reporting suspected adverse drug reactions	123

Last Words	125
Campaigning for Change	126
Resources	129
Organisations	129
Ombudsmen	131
Websites and Links	132
Maternity Policies	133
Books	134
References	137

Foreword

There are many fine examples of exemplary maternity care in both the UK and elsewhere. These examples happen because of the midwives and other practitioners who are passionate about providing the care they were trained to give, and want to provide, to women, babies and families. They know that it matters to women, and that it can be transformatory, to be listened to and to be supported to make their own decisions about their pregnancies, births and babies.

Committed, skilled midwives support women to birth as straightforwardly as possible, watchfully waiting, quietly encouraging, helping women to stay calm and focused, and offering to use low tech midwifery skills only when these will help the birthing woman and her baby and avoid the need for further more invasive interventions. If complications arise, they are able to refer women to obstetricians. Many women are particularly vulnerable during childbearing, and midwives and other practitioners in some areas have set up services with the specific aim of providing the kind of culturally and socially sensitive care and continuity that enables these women to make decisions about pregnancy and birth and during the postnatal period.

Overall, however, routine and potentially harmful interventions and obstetric technology are over-used throughout many parts of the world (Brownlee et al 2017, Seijmonsbergen-Schermer et al 2019). This makes for wide variability within maternity services. Maternity care can even vary within the same area or hospital. A recent online survey of 1,145 women, through the organisations Mumsnet and Birthrights in the UK, reported that 14% of the women said that their plans for birth were overruled and that for a further 11% there were attempts to overrule their decisions for birth. Overall, 24% of the mothers surveyed said that their decisions and views were not respected and 30% said their views were not asked for at all (www.birthrights.org.uk). While this survey was relatively small and self-selecting, it is worrying nonetheless.

Globally, women's rights and decisions are regularly overridden and some women continue to receive disrespectful care. Sometimes this amounts to obstetric violence (UN Report 2019). For example, in one

European country a woman was subjected to multiple vaginal examinations, induction of labour, episiotomy and forceps without her consent. She successfully appealed to the United Nations Committee on the Elimination of Discrimination against Women on the grounds that her rights had been violated. In 2018, the Committee found in her favour and ordered that she should receive compensation. It also required the hospital staff to introduce staff training on women's rights, and conduct studies to reveal the extent of obstetric violence in that country. Similar appeals from three other women have yet to be heard.

We know that for black and Asian women, their risk of dying during childbearing in the UK and Ireland is nearly five and nearly two times greater respectively than white women (MBRRACE-UK 2019), and while it will take more than human rights legislation to improve their outcomes and those of their babies, these can play a part. We know that for women living in poverty, and for those women who have received less formal education, their voices are not as easily sought or heard as the voices of more affluent women (Lindquist et al 2014, Rance et al 2013). We know too, that some of these women are more likely to receive avoidable interventions. For these women, changes in the structure of maternity care, cultural biases and communication are needed if they are to be enabled to make the decisions they wish to.

For some women, their rights during birth may seem less meaningful, and very much more difficult to assert, when they are struggling with pressing matters such as homelessness, poverty, racism, intimate violence and other life difficulties. Inequalities of any kind impact on how much we can draw on human rights, in the same way that they impact on every other aspect of our lives.

Why women's decisions are not always asked for, respected or acted upon, and why technology is so prevalent, is not the main topic of this book, but it might be useful to have some understanding about this. Many activists, sociologists, researchers and others have addressed these challenging questions. While the reasons are complex, they generally agree that numbers of influential strands have contributed to this, such as how women and reproductive processes are viewed in society; the growth of and dependence on science and technology (which, despite its flaws and side effects, results in the assumption that only further science and technology will provide answers and better outcomes); the focus on risk and its management (so while childbirth is safer than ever for women and babies in the UK and other well-resourced countries, fear is pervasive, and when adverse outcomes occur, blame is often attributed to the women and/or those caring for her); and the destabilising of health care services (where they and other public services have been increasingly starved of resources, centralised, standardised and bound by rules). Practitioners are, therefore, often providing care in a context of too little time to engage with people they have never met before, too heavy a workload, little support from colleagues or managers, and a fear that if anything goes wrong and they have not followed the 'rules', they will be blamed. In this kind of environment it can be difficult, if not impossible, for midwives to support women and difficult for women to resist routine interventions. It is, in addition, unconducive to women feeling calm, relaxed, and confident enough to enable their birth hormones to flow and their births to unfold in their own time and ways. Good relational based care from empathic, engaged practitioners happens despite, rather than because of, the way the maternity services are currently organised (Reed 2020).

As Beverley rightly emphasises, one of the best known ways to support women's decisions and to improve outcomes for mothers and babies is to introduce the continuity of maternity care recommended by the four UK governments. Research from all over the world has unequivocally shown that all women and babies have better outcomes, less intervention, and are more satisfied with their care, when they receive continuity of midwifery care from skilled midwives who are well-resourced, well supported and have autonomy over their work patterns.

Given the current context, however, normal birth without interventions and out of hospital births are relatively less common in the UK and other high income countries. Thus, this book provides extensive sections about normal birth and home birth, and the rights women have when planning and/or having these, so that they might have the best chance of having as straightforward a birth as possible. This is not to say that normal birth or home birth is best for all women and babies: clearly, some women and babies require obstetric and other expertise and technology and would not survive or do well without these, physically and/or emotionally. In some cases, and in some parts of the world, women who need obstetric technology have no access to it or have it withheld (Miller et al 2016). Thus, knowing about rights is important for women whatever their circumstances and decisions.

It is also important to be aware of our rights because these are not set in stone and can be strengthened or eroded, depending on the specific political and environmental landscape at the time. During the first wave of the COVID-19 pandemic for example, some of the rights that women normally have during childbearing were suspended. These were usually suspended temporarily, to protect the NHS from being overwhelmed and to protect practitioners and those using the services. Human rights, however, cannot be easily put aside and sometimes the measures taken were considered to be disproportionate and, in some countries, the suspension of women's rights does not appear to be temporary (Drandic and Leeuwen 2020). Unless we know what rights women have, we cannot make sure that they are reinstated at the first possible moment, or continue to build on and strengthen them.

Beverley has supported thousands of women during her long career as a maternity activist. Writing from many years of research and experience, she sets out very clearly women's basic rights during childbearing. She gives many examples of the kinds of decisions women in many of the high income countries might face during this time, and their rights to make the best decisions for them, their babies, and families. Of course, her book can only cover general principles and typical examples. These will apply differently to different women, and policies and practices will vary from region to region and country to country.

Many women are unlikely to need this book, but may still want to know what their rights are out of interest or in case they find themselves in a situation where they need to know and assert these. For those women who find that their decisions are being questioned or potentially overridden, it will be an invaluable resource.

Nadine Pilley Edwards

Drandic, Daniela and van Leeuwen, Fleur (2020) 'But a Small Price to Pay – Degredation of Rights in Childbirth During COVID-19. (OxHRH Blog, April 2020), ohrh.law.ox.ac.uk/but-a-small-price-to-pay-degradation-of-rights-in-childbirth-during-covid-19/, [Accessed 6 Feb 2021].

My Experience of Maternity Care

As a fit and healthy 27-year-old woman expecting my first baby, I had an uneventful pregnancy and gave up my work as an administrator in the Ministry of Defence four weeks before my baby was due. As advised, I went into hospital when the contractions were coming every five minutes, where I and my husband were ushered by a midwife into a room. I climbed onto the bed, and before long the contractions stopped. A midwife arrived and informed me that they would be setting up a drip to *"get me going"*. Naively, I accepted this as a thought went through my mind, *"oh yes, they mentioned induction at antenatal classes."*

Thirty-six hours later, still wired up to the drip and a fetal monitor (the final print-out was almost a foot high), after a failed epidural, flat on my back with my feet in stirrups, my 9lb 10oz son arrived. His birth was assisted by Neville Barnes forceps, which are used for delivering babies who are in a normal, head down position. He was held up by his heels and flopped like a piece of wet fish as they whisked him over to a resuscitaire. I lay there thinking, *"Have I gone through all this to give birth to a dead baby?"*

One of the paediatricians came over to me, held my hand, and said, *"It is all right, your baby is fine."* On reflection, I came to realise that although I suffered postnatal depression for about 18 months, her action saved me from having post-traumatic stress. Over the next ten days, the only person who acknowledged my awful birth experience was the ward cleaner who said, *"You have had a really tough time love."* My son stayed in special care until I limped in some days later and demanded my baby. The midwife's reaction was, *"Oh, he is such a lovely baby, the biggest one we have had."* I wondered why he was there and suspected he need not have been.

Over the next few months I slowly recovered, physically if not mentally. I kept going over in my head why I was the only woman who could not birth a baby easily, and how I had gone into hospital a fit and healthy young woman, but had come out a physical and mental wreck. Eventually I decided to seek an appointment with my obstetrician,

Am I Allowed: 4th Edition

Stanley Simmons, who had not come near me all the time I was in hospital. I could not get an appointment, so I wrote to Ronald Bell, then the Member of Parliament for Buckinghamshire. When writing asking for an MP's help I was advised to give all the information I had, so the poor man was subjected to four pages of a blow-by-blow account of my labour and birth.

I got an appointment with Stanley within a week, ironically, nine months after the birth. By this time, having gone over and over in my head every aspect of the birth, and bored my husband and just about everyone else stiff, I was ready. In floods of tears, I grilled Stanley for over an hour about the birth, and soon realised that he was not going to answer my questions. He kept patting the foot-high pile of fetal monitoring traces saying, *"I would be proud to show these records to anyone."* He was worried that I was going to sue. I said, *"I don't care who you show them to."* I was not interested in taking legal action. I wanted answers, so I asked the killer question: *"There was no clinical reason whatsoever for my labour to be induced, was there?"* He simply stared at me. I had my answer.

Over the next couple of years I talked to women in the village about their birth experiences. They all appeared happy and healthy, but as I spoke with them, their birth stories emerged, and I realised that some of them had had even worse experiences than me, and it was then that I got angry. How could this hidden trauma be allowed to happen? That was when I embarked on a new career - campaigning for change in maternity services.

The wonderful Jean Robinson, who was President of the Patients' Association at the time, and went on to become President of the Association for Improvements in the Maternity Services (AIMS) until her resignation in 2017, had written an article in *The Times* about the overuse of induction of labour. I wrote to her asking her to write another article about how to get over the experience. At the end of my letter I said that I wanted to do something to change what was happening.

She wrote back advising me to join AIMS, which I did. A year later, in 1977, I was elected Honorary Chair. Forty years later, in 2017, I resigned from that position but the campaign continues because, for example, women still struggle to assert their rights in maternity care and intervention rates have increased dramatically, with births by caesarean surgery going from fewer than 10% in the 1970s to over 30% in many large obstetric units today, with no corresponding improvement in the health of mothers and babies.

Am I Allowed: 4th Edition

ACRONYMS USED IN THIS BOOK

ABM	Association of Breastfeeding Mothers
AIMS	Association for Improvements in the Maternity Services
AIS	Adverse Incidents Scotland
AMU	Alongside Midwifery Unit
ARM	Artificial Rupture of Membranes
AvMA	Action against Medical Accidents
BAPM	British Association of Perinatal Medicine
CHC	Community Health Council
CTG	Cardiotocography (Electronic Fetal Monitoring)
CVS	Chorionic Villus Sampling
EFM	Electronic Fetal Monitoring
FMU	Free-standing Midwifery Unit
GBS	Group B Streptococcus
GDPR	General Data Protection Regulation
GP	General Practitioner
Hb	Haemoglobin
HBAC	Home Birth after a Caesarean
HIV	Human Immunodeficiency Virus
HPs	Health Practitioners - doctors midwives, nurses or health visitors
MDU	Medical Defence Union
MHRA	Medicines and Healthcare Products Regulatory Agency
NHS	National Health Service
NICE	National Institute for Health and Care Excellence
NMPA	National Maternity and Perinatal Audit
NRLS	National Reporting and Learning System
OU	Consultant or Obstetric Unit
PALS	Patient Advice and Liaison Services
PHE	Public Health England
PTSD	Post Traumatic Stress Disorder
RCOG	Royal College of Obstetricians and Gynaecologists
RCPCH	Royal College of Paediatrics and Child Health
SANDS	Stillbirth and Neonatal Death Society
UK	United Kingdom
VBAC	Vaginal Birth After Caesarean
VE	Vaginal Examination
WHICH?	A consumer campaigning organisation
WHO	World Health Organization

Introduction

One of the most common questions I have been asked over the years is "am I allowed?" So many women think that they have to do as they are told by others, not realising that it is their body and their baby, and they are the ones who have the right to say yes or no to any intervention. Health Professionals (HPs) have a duty to explain why they want to carry out a particular procedure and to provide detailed information about its possible benefits and harms, but if women do not agree they have an absolute right to decline.

This book is intended to inform you about the kind of maternity services available, to help you make decisions about the kind of maternity care you want, and to help you understand what rights you have in maternity care, so that you can start thinking about the right decisions for you and your baby, maybe even before you embark on your first pregnancy.

You may well not be faced with the kinds of issues I address in this book, but I believe in the principle that it is better to be properly informed so that, if you are, you are well prepared. For many women there will be no problems, but if there are, at least you will have the information you need to be able to make decisions that are best for you and your baby.

This revised edition of *Am I Allowed?* comes at a time of a potentially huge change in maternity service provision, and during the restrictions caused by Covid-19 (see Chapter 2).

All four countries in the UK have produced plans to improve maternity services so that women have real choice of continuity of midwifery care and where to give birth (see Resources, Maternity Policies). We are, however, still living with over-medicalised birth and fragmented services, and few of the targets made by various Government reports, have been met.

NHS maternity statistics for England released in October 2019 showed that spontaneous onset of labour has decreased *"from 69% in 2008-09 to 50% in 2018-19"* and a *"Caesarean method of onset increased from 11% to 17% and induced method of onset from 20% to 22% in the period*

2008-09 -2018-19." (NHS Digital 2019). Unfortunately, these figures do not include those women who had emergency caesareans or accelerated labours.

This has resulted in many women being processed through a system that relies on overly rigid protocols, tick boxes, and too many unnecessary interventions, irrespective of the evidence that there are better outcomes and satisfaction for both women and midwives when the women receive continuity of midwifery care.

Furthermore, the Royal College of Midwives survey (Downe and Finlayson 2016) in England showed that: *"25% of births recorded as normal involved artificial rupture of membranes and 22% included induction of labour."*

Maternity services have been so starved of resources and practitioners so over-burdened and demoralised that it is increasingly challenging for them to provide the care they are trained for and want to provide (Kirkham 2019).

Despite this, there are many midwives who work both in hospitals and in communities who care deeply about supporting women's decision-making and who provide excellent midwifery care. There are skilled doctors who provide sensitive obstetric care where it is needed, so that however birth unfolds, women are able to look back on their births with joy and satisfaction.

The National Health Service (NHS) provides maternity services for the majority of women in the UK. Many women are unaware that they have rights and options within that system. When women first become pregnant, they sometimes struggle to know what maternity services are available, or where they could go to obtain good quality information or care.

Unfortunately, the hundreds of books and magazines on pregnancy and childbirth often don't give you information that will enable you to weigh up your options, so that you can make informed decisions. Research has shown, however, that many women assume without good information that the care on offer must *"be best"* (Teijlingen et al 2003) and, therefore, they usually accept whatever is recommended, on the grounds that it must be safe, and assume that it must be effective or health professionals (HPs) would not be using it, and women might not know what questions to ask.

While many policies and practices have changed over recent years, some NHS publications still seem to be designed to accustom women to the policies and practices generally in use. On the surface these appear to offer choice, but there can be an implicit expectation that women will comply.

The media is increasingly used as the main source of information about birth. This often reflects a particular view of birth. For example, One Born Every Minute (OBEM), a popular and heavily edited television programme in the UK and other countries, sensationalises the reality of birth in large obstetric units and without commenting on the poor care and inappropriate interventions that it often reveals. OBEM makes no comment on the high level of interventions the women receive, and an article analysing the content of this kind of programme found that informed choice was lacking (De Benedictis et al 2018). The programme gives the impression that birth is a painful ordeal to be endured, and obscures the fact that this is often a result of various interventions, and a lack of support from a known and trusted midwife who is supported by a system that enables her to use her midwifery skills and knowledge. Gentle, tranquil, and straightforward normal births do not make exciting viewing.

Fortunately, to redress the balance, in recent years there has been a growing number of informative books, mainly written by experienced midwives and lay people (see Resources, Books).

While acknowledging that there are male midwives currently practising, throughout this book I have referred to midwives as *she*, thereby avoiding as much as possible the rather clumsy s/he or her/him, and rather than mention doctor, midwife, nurse or health visitor each time I have referred to them as health professionals (HPs).

In this book, I have included Chapter 10 – When Things Don't Go to Plan. Some people feel that it is not appropriate to include discussion of adverse events in books for pregnant women; but if we do not include such discussions then the parents who may have a problem, and who most need support and information, may not know where to turn. I believe that it is better to be well informed, but if you do not agree you can always skip that chapter.

Where older research has been cited, this is because no new research has been done to challenge or substantiate its findings.

This book does not cover employment rights (see Resources, Organisations). It focuses primarily on the maternity rights of parents in the UK, but much of the information is also appropriate for those in other high income countries. In many of these, women's rights in reproduction have been acknowledged, to a greater or lesser extent, but many women across the world struggle to have these recognised, or acted upon, and in many places these hard won rights are being eroded.

This book is intended to inform you about the kind of maternity services available, to help you make decisions about the kind of maternity care you want, and to help you understand what rights you have in maternity care, so that you can make the right decisions for you and your baby, maybe even before you embark on your first pregnancy.

You may well not be faced with the kinds of issues I address in this book, but if you are, this book will help you be well prepared and, however your pregnancy and birth unfold, you will have the information you need to be able to make decisions that are best for you and your baby.

Chapter 1
The Complexities of Choice

A little bit of history

In the UK, AIMS was the first organisation to campaign on women's human rights, although at that time it was simply referred to as women's rights. Since then, Birthrights and the White Ribbon Alliance have been established, by lawyers and birth activists, to promote respect for human rights in childbirth in the UK and internationally (see Resources, Organisations).

Over the years, battles have been fought to have women's rights established and respected. However, in the current climate of fear and litigation, standardised services, high levels of intervention and too few midwives, if you make decisions outside a hospital's guidelines or routines, you can face difficulties.

Early on in my role as Honorary Chair of AIMS, I was dismayed by the general belief that pregnant and birthing women had to do what the doctors wanted, and in looking for reasons for this belief I came across a Medical Defence Union (MDU) statement in a booklet, which said:

"The Union does not consider that a maternity patient need give her written consent to any operative or manipulative procedures that are normally associated with childbirth. When she enters hospital for her confinement it can be assumed that she assents to any necessary procedure, including the administration of a local, general or other anaesthetic." (Medical Defence Union, 1974).

Some hospitals even printed this statement on the inside cover of women's case notes. In 1979, I wrote to the MDU asking for a copy of the law, regulation or statute which allowed it to make this statement. No-one ever replied to my letter, but the statement was withdrawn from the next booklet. While the withdrawal of this statement implied an acceptance of a woman's right to agree or decline treatment, the attitude that the doctors had a right to dictate persisted.

Am I Allowed: 4th Edition

On the 4th April 1982 a demonstration was attended by over 5,000 people, to protest at the policy of an obstetrician at the Royal Free Hospital in London, who insisted that all women must birth on their backs, on a bed. During the demonstration, a colleague and activist, Patricia Barki, suggested that AIMS should organise a petition demanding that women's rights in maternity care be written into law. My attempts to find out precisely what rights women had, involved a lot of searching. I realised that if we were to present a petition then we should properly inform the MPs of the problems. That is how I ended up writing *Denial of Parents' Rights in Maternity Care* for AIMS in 1983. It was not long before I received letters asking for a copy and, finally, it dawned on me that the reason women were asking for copies was because they did not know what rights they did have. That booklet ultimately became the book you are reading now.

Over the years, attitudes to pregnant and labouring women have gradually changed. There is increasing acknowledgement that women have the right to determine what care they will have, who will attend them, and where they will give birth.

Doctors and midwives are very much more aware nowadays that it is your body and your baby, and that they are not entitled to carry out any treatment without your consent. Obviously, for some of the routine procedures (such as taking a blood sample), you may not be asked, in words of one syllable, for your consent. The HP will assume, for example, that rolling up your sleeve and presenting your arm is sufficient indication that you are prepared to have a blood sample taken. Some practitioners still mistakenly believe that consent will always be given if they give enough information and give it to you correctly.

It is, however, your body and your baby and you are the one who makes the decisions. HPs are required to make sure that you have good information based on available evidence and that you understand it. Then they must respect your decision.

Choice and decision making

NHS England's 5 Year Plan (2016) for improving maternity services requires that women have *"Personalised care, centred on the woman, her baby and her family, based around their needs and their decisions, where they have genuine choice, informed by unbiased information."* (National Maternity Review 2016).

Similar statements have been made by the Health and Social Care Board in Northern Ireland and by the Scottish and Welsh Governments.

Women's choices and decision-making, however, are influenced by hospital guidelines that they rarely see. These are general guidelines which focus on a one size fits all approach. They cannot focus on the individual, they are not always based on robust evidence and often balance evidence with economics; they are what they say they are – guidelines only.

While practice remains variable across regions and countries, in many countries it is not uncommon for women to be told that they must do this, or they must do that, or that the hospital's guidelines have to be followed. You may be told things like:
"I will book you in at the clinic ..."
"You will have to see the consultant"
"You have to have this test"
"I've made an appointment for your scan next week"
"We don't allow women to go over 40 weeks"

As a result, you, like many women, may become anxious and concerned. Your feeling sometimes tells you that you do not want to *comply* – it's just not right for me, or my baby. For example, you might ask: *"Am I allowed to refuse an induction or a scan?"*

The answer to that question is YES! You are. It's your body and your baby, and as with any other medical test or procedure, you have a right to say no, and you should not have to say it more than once. The assumption that *one size fits all* does not recognise that it might not be right for an individual woman and her baby. You have a right to see the guidelines and a right not to follow them. Sara Wickham's book *What's*

Right For Me? (2018) is an excellent guide to decision making, and Amy Brown's book *Informed is Best* (2019) is a guide to help you evaluate evidence and information to enable you to come to a decision that is right for you and your baby.

Coercing you into accepting treatment you do not want constitutes obstetric violence and is an assault. Many women who have been persuaded into agreeing to something they were not happy about find this difficult to live with.

There is much emphasis on *choice* in the maternity services. This usually means offering a predetermined menu, such as a Birth Plan, from which you can choose, rather than discussing the options with you and encouraging you to write your own birth plan.

Although written in 2006, Dr Allmark's observations are still relevant today. *"We are developing a culture of conformity which pays lip service to autonomy and choice but within which the individual is only really free to make the choice that is approved by the state. It is assumed that once the 'healthy choice' is pointed out, everyone will select it and no account is taken of the very differing circumstances and aspirations of different people's lives."* (Allmark 2006).

Even decision making is being undermined by the current focus on *shared decision making*. This suggests that HPs and women share the decision. This is not so. It is your decision, and yours alone. A rare exception, for example, may be a woman who can be shown to *lack mental capacity* (see Birthrights 2017).

Sometimes you may be told that it is hospital policy for a particular intervention to be offered at a particular point in your labour, but not all women and babies are the same, and you may be one of those women for whom the intervention will not be of benefit. As Nadine Edwards explains in her book *Birthing Your Baby* (2019) there are uncertainties and limitations to research and it may not necessarily apply to you.

Doctors and midwives, who are invariably busy, and who rarely encounter women who decline tests and interventions, may assume that your consent has been given, or wrongly believe that they can/should overrule your decision, or coerce you to follow their advice *"for the safety of the fetus"* (Kruske et al 2013) because they are concerned that they will be held responsible if an adverse outcome occurs. Some practitioners, despite carefully documenting that they are respecting and supporting a woman's decision, have been unjustly disciplined, further complicating decision-making. This can make it even more difficult for women to make their own decisions and for practitioners to support them.

The issue of *informed refusal* is yet to be addressed adequately, or even generally understood. The NHS has made a very clear statement on this: *"If you refuse a treatment, your decision must be respected, even if [it] is thought that refusing treatment would result in your death or the death of your unborn child."* (NHS 2017).

Sometimes some HPs need reminding of this statement.

Guidelines

Hospital policies and practices are based on guidelines and every maternity unit produces policies and guidelines for the management of childbirth. Many of them will be based on National Institute for Health and Care Excellence (NICE) and Royal College of Obstetricians and Gynaecologists (RCOG) Guidelines. These are based on available research evidence, and where such evidence is unavailable it is based on the opinion of experienced practitioners. They have been developed to aid clinicians in undertaking what is thought to be best practice, so the procedures on offer, or carried out, should be based on these. Even so, not all hospital guidelines are based on robust research evidence (Prusova et al 2014). Sometimes this is because no well-conducted trials have been undertaken, and not all hospital guidelines are updated when new knowledge becomes available.

In 1979, Professor Archie Cochrane awarded obstetrics a wooden spoon for being the least evidence-based medical speciality. There have been many improvements since then but, nevertheless, many routine interventions in maternity care are not appropriate for every woman.

If you are concerned about the proposals for your care, and unsure about precisely what interventions will be offered in labour, you are entitled to ask for a copy of the guidelines that relate to your particular circumstances. For example, if you intend having a vaginal birth after a caesarean (VBAC), or you are expecting twins, or your baby is presenting by the breech, you can ask for a copy of the relevant guidelines for the proposed management of labour.

Finally, guidelines are there to guide HPs. They are not rules that you have to agree with or that the care giver has to abide by.

You have a right to ask questions, a right to ask for a second opinion, and a right to decline treatment and await developments should you wish.

Your decisions and the responsibilities of the midwife

Before making a decision you may have carefully researched the medical evidence, your options, and the implications for your care. You also have your own knowledge of your body, of your growing baby, and of family traits, such as family stories of babies who rarely arrive before 43 weeks.

You may know the exact date when you conceived, contrary to what the ultrasound determined. This knowledge is often ignored, undermined, or dismissed, in the discussion about the *right choice* by some HPs who believe that they know better but are, if fact, treating women like children.

Some HPs automatically presume that a woman who declines their advice puts her baby at risk and is behaving irresponsibly. If, however, a baby has problems during or following a birth, the mother can be perceived, in retrospect, as having taken the *wrong* decision, based on an assumption that a different course of action would have made a difference; and many of those who have problems following an induction or a caesarean will be faced with an assumption that, despite the problems, the *right* decision was made.

When a HP talks about a woman *taking full responsibility* this implies that she is making the *wrong choice*. Furthermore, making a decision to go against medical advice does not absolve the HPs should there be any negligence on their part.

Occasionally, a HP suggests that if a woman persists with her decision her baby could die. While this is possible in certain circumstances, and you need to know the benefits and risks of what you plan, this is unethical, unacceptable, and against practitioners' Codes of Practice when used coercively. For example, midwives are expected to: *"respect, support and document a person's right to accept or refuse care and treatment."* (Nursing and Midwifery Council 2015).

Birth Plans

Many women now choose to complete birth plans; these plans were first proposed by the UK's Association of Radical Midwives and originally called *A Letter to the Midwife*, because the midwives were concerned that women were receiving interventions that they did not necessarily need or want. Whether or not you write a formal birth plan and share it with your midwife and others, it can be a useful way of thinking through what's important to you and discussing this with your birth partner/s. Birth plans can also be very helpful for midwives who are striving to support your decisions, or for partners or doulas to draw the HP's attention to what you want, especially if the HPs are not listening to what you are saying.

If you decide to write a birth plan you may find it helpful to begin by stating that you have thought carefully about the issues, and that you would appreciate support from the midwives to achieve the kind of birth you want. You may well find that the majority of midwives will react positively to such a statement.

One difficulty is that birth plans that have been devised by hospitals tend to highlight the choices that the hospital provides and may not give much information about the implications of these, nor information about any alternatives. To assist you in thinking through what you want, Sara Wickham, in 2018, published the second edition of *What's Right For*

Am I Allowed: 4th Edition

Me? which is designed to help you consider your options before completing your birth plan and finalising your decisions, and Milli Hill's *The Positive Birth Book Visual Birth Plan Cards* (2020) can be used to help you decide what you want to include in your birth plan.

Chapter 2

Planning Ahead: Who Will Attend You?

Considering your options

Planning your maternity care will involve three different questions: who will care for me?; what kind of care would I like to receive?; and where would I like to give birth? These options are usually inter-related, so it is important to consider beforehand what kind of birth you are hoping for before you make a decision. If you are planning to have a normal, physiological birth, without medical interventions, the maternity services you choose will influence whether or not you are more likely to achieve this.

It cannot be stressed enough that many women in the UK receive excellent maternity care from practitioners who work tirelessly to focus on them, their aspirations and their individual circumstances. They do everything they can to make sure that the women in their care receive the support they need and to ensure that their decisions are respected, even when these fall outside usual policies and practices.

There are many examples of senior midwives spending time with women, and liaising with midwifery and medical colleagues, to make sure that they are well supported and their decisions respected. One senior midwife told us that she spends a great deal of her time with women making decisions in complex situations. Her conversations always start with: *"We will support you with whatever choices you make and the reason for our meeting is so that I can ensure you have access to and understand the best available evidence we have, recognise the limitations of that evidence, and the opportunity to ask questions so that you are making a fully informed, non-biased choice without any judgement from a professional."*

The implications of Covid-19

During the height of the Covid-19 pandemic, health services responded differently throughout the UK and across the globe. Women's rights to determine where to birth, and who to have with them, were seriously challenged (Drandić and Leeuwen 2020), despite there being little evidence to support many of the restrictions imposed in maternity care. In some areas, home births were suspended and midwifery units were closed, while in others, home births and birth in midwifery units were deemed to be safer and encouraged. In many areas, services have been largely restored, but remain variable.

In other areas, women were initially restricted to one or no companions in labour, but as time passed this ruling was relaxed. Indeed, the RCOG/RCM guidance states that: *"Women should be permitted and encouraged to have a birth partner present with them in their labour and during birth. Having a trusted birth partner present throughout labour is known to make a significant difference to the safety and well-being of women in childbirth."* (RCOG/RCM 2020).

The Royal College of Paediatrics and Child Health (RCPCH) has stated that: *"Healthy babies born to suspected/confirmed Covid19 mothers and who do not require medical intervention should remain with their mother in their designated room."* (RCPCH 2020).

As Government and local guidelines can still change on a weekly or even daily basis, you can consult Covid-19 guidelines and restrictions nationally and locally for up-to-date information, and contact one of the support groups if you have any concerns (see Organisations – page 129).

Choosing your birth supporters

The following are the main professionals who might be involved in your care, and your rights in relation to them.

Every woman in the UK has the right to be attended by an NHS midwife during pregnancy, birth and postnatally, whatever her circumstances. Women who are unsure about whether or not they are entitled to free

NHS care can contact AIMS, or Maternity Action (see Resources, Organisations).

Due to additional responsibilities, shortages of midwives in many areas and an emphasis on efficiency, many midwives are less able to provide the emotional support and relational care that they used to, and still want to, give.

Antenatal classes have significantly reduced; there are fewer, they cover less ground and, if you have had a baby before, there is even less provision. Over the years, postnatal care has become a shadow of that which was provided 40 years ago.

The majority of NHS midwives work in large, centralised obstetric units, alongside, or within, free-standing midwifery units, or in the community. While midwifery education and training enable midwives to support birth, and provide continuity of care, this can often be difficult in a medically dominated system. Despite these constraints, the majority of NHS midwives do their best to support women and respond to their needs, and many hospitals are now providing for midwives and obstetricians to train together and appreciate each other's skills and expertise. In some areas, for example, senior midwives and obstetricians have created dedicated teams to support women having vaginal breech births.

Some women who find their local service unresponsive to their needs seek the support of a doula, and a small number of women contact an independent or private midwife.

An independent/private midwife is fully qualified, registered with the Nursing and Midwifery Council, and usually specialises in supporting normal birth at home, but since increased insurance requirements the numbers of independent/private midwives have reduced significantly and some areas have no independent or private midwives.

A doula is usually engaged directly by you to provide emotional support during labour, although many hospitals are now recruiting doulas. Though not always the case, this can mean that the doula's main responsibility is to the hospital and its rules, rather than you. A Cochrane Review found that having a supporter who is not a HP with you increases your chances of having a spontaneous vaginal birth (Bohren et al 2017).

You have the right to decide who will be with you during labour, and this can include husbands, partners, relatives, friends and/or doulas, but see local guidelines on this during the Covid-19 pandemic. In normal circumstances, you have the right to insist that your choice of companion remains with you.

Midwives

Midwives are experts in normal pregnancy, labour and birth and refer women who need additional help to an obstetrician or other relevant specialists. You have the right to book with a midwife for your maternity services directly.

In recent years, with the centralisation of birth into large obstetric units, many midwives are less able to develop the skills they need to attend and support a normal birth, unless they are working in a Free-standing Midwifery Unit (FMU), Birth Centre, or are part of a community home birth team.

NHS midwifery services differ from area to area. For example, in some areas care is provided by a team of community midwives. These teams can vary in size from four to 20 midwives and mainly offer an antenatal and postnatal service; most women go into hospital for birth and are looked after by labour ward midwives. In other areas, midwives work in the community in small groups, and carry their own caseloads of women. These midwives provide continuity of carer antenatally, during labour and birth, and postnatally, wherever a woman has her baby.

Research has shown that this kind of care is very beneficial (Sandall et al 2016) as women are:

"16% less likely to lose their baby
19% less likely to lose their baby before 24 weeks
16% less likely to have an episiotomy
and:
15% fewer had an epidural or spinal

*10% fewer had their waters broken
and there were:
10% fewer instrumental deliveries (forceps or ventouse)
24% fewer pre-term births"*

The evidence also shows that women who had midwife-led continuity of care were more likely to have a spontaneous vaginal birth (Sandall et al 2016). Recent research shows that *"caseload midwifery outperforms standard care in perceived quality of pregnancy care regardless of risk."* (Allen 2019). You can ask if this way of working is available in your area, and if not, why not.

"Women will experience continuity of carer across the whole of their maternity journey." (Welsh Government 2019). Similar sentiments have been expressed from the English (2016), Scottish (2017) and Northern Irish (2012) governments.

Consultant midwives

Consultant midwives are senior midwives with an advanced level of clinical midwifery expertise. They are usually based in a maternity unit and have a lead role in midwifery education, training and development. They often have a wide range of experience in supporting women whose decisions do not comply with hospital guidance; women who have had previous difficult births; and women who have other specific needs. Any woman can approach them for advice and support.

Private/independent midwifery care

You may choose to engage a private/independent midwife. Women who have had traumatic births previously and want to give themselves the best chance of avoiding a repetition sometimes seek the care of an independent midwife. Others want to be attended by a midwife they know, which is not common in NHS services; others want to give themselves the best chance of a normal birth and feel that they stand a better chance of achieving that with a private/independent midwife that they have been able to get to know and trust.

Private Midwives

Private Midwives is a company that offers midwives a contract of employment, giving them employment practice privileges or, alternatively, the opportunity to be covered by PRISM (Professional Risk and Indemnity Scheme for Midwives). The midwives are fully qualified and offer continuity of midwifery care at home or in an NHS hospital. They tend to specialise in normal physiological birth and offer individualised care to a small number of women, but are constrained by their insurance company's restrictions, compared with NHS midwives who may be restricted by routines and practices and large caseloads. Like their NHS colleagues, they are registered with and regulated by the Nursing and Midwifery Council (see Resources, Organisations).

Independent midwives

Independent Midwives UK are also fully qualified midwives who offer antenatal and postnatal care, work directly with families, and can be booked directly by women and their families.

At present, as a result of the Nursing and Midwifery Council's ruling that all midwives practising outside the NHS must be covered by commercial indemnity insurance, and the Royal College of Midwives decision only to provide indemnity insurance for NHS employed midwives, *Independent Midwives UK* is seeking to raise sufficient money to provide insurance cover for intrapartum (during birth) care.

Booking an independent midwife is not dependent upon the approval of your NHS midwife, GP or obstetrician, and it does not take away any entitlement to use NHS maternity services. Interestingly, during the Covid-19 epidemic some hospitals arranged contracts with independent midwives to provide antenatal, intrapartum and postnatal care so they could help cover the increased demand for home births (see Resources, Organisations).

General Practitioner (GP) services

It is now unusual for women to have *shared maternity care* from a GP and a midwife. Of course, you can see your GP at any point during or after pregnancy for health concerns such as, for example, a sore toe or a chest infection.

Overall, GPs have become less involved with maternity services and if approached will most likely refer you to your local midwife or to a local consultant obstetrician. In some areas, however, some GPs have recently become re-involved in antenatal care and GP practices still provide a 6-week postnatal check for mother and baby.

Obstetric services

Obstetricians are specialist doctors who care for women with pregnancy and birth related medical problems. If you have health problems, or problems during your pregnancy, or have had difficulties during previous pregnancies or births, you should be referred for a consultation with an obstetrician and/or an appropriate specialist.

Some hospitals, however, routinely book all women under obstetric care, despite the majority being fit and healthy who should, more appropriately, be receiving midwifery care only, with the option of being referred to an obstetrician if, or when, needed or wanted.

While not all obstetricians share a medicalised view of birth and some provide a woman-focused service, overall they are more likely than midwives to recommend interventions.

Am I Allowed: 4th Edition

Health visitor services

Health visitors are registered nurses and/or midwives who have additional training in community public health nursing. They offer support and advice after your baby has been born until your child is five years old. They are usually based in children's centres, GP surgeries, community or health centres. In most areas health visitors are introduced to you antenatally, so that you will know that there is a health visitor available after your baby is born. Their services are offered to every pregnant woman, as the NHS has a duty to provide a service for new mothers and their children beyond the midwifery service. Some women appreciate the health visitor's offer of help and support, but others do not feel the need for this extra input and you can choose to decline their involvement.

You are under no obligation whatsoever to see, or admit, a health visitor into your home if you do not want to. Health visitors do not have a right of access to your home.

Medical and/or midwifery student services

Whether you birth at home or in hospital you may be asked to agree to the attendance and participation of a midwifery and/or medical student. They are often keen to learn and most women find them very supportive. Some women, however, are made anxious by the presence of yet another person. You have the right to refuse to be watched or attended by a medical, midwifery, nursing, health visiting or any other student, and your permission should always be sought.

Second opinion

If you are concerned about the advice that you are being given, or the treatment proposed, either for you or your baby, you have a right to a second opinion. If you have difficulty getting one you could approach the hospital's Consultant Midwife or the Director/Head of Midwifery. They should be listed on the local hospital's web site, or you can contact your local or national support groups for information (see Resources, organisations). You might want to ask to be referred to a HP in a different hospital, or check locally to see whether there is a HP who would be more supportive of your decisions/preferences.

Changing your service provider

The majority of midwives, general practitioners, obstetricians, health visitors and other HPs are conscientious and hard-working individuals who are doing their best to give you the best possible care.

Occasionally, for whatever reason, you may wish to change your HP. Should you not be happy with a particular person attending you at any time, including in labour, you have a right to refuse to be looked after by them, and they have a duty to find you another HP, even if you are giving birth at home.

Changing your midwife

Once in a while, a woman finds that she is not happy with her midwife and would like to see someone different. Midwives acknowledge that not everyone gets on with everyone else, so there should be no problem in changing your midwife. You can either let her know that you would prefer to be seen by someone else or, if she is not happy to facilitate a change, you can contact your local Director/Head of Midwifery. You may wish to explain why you want to change, but you do not have to give a reason.

Some years ago, a woman contacted me asking how to change her midwife. She explained that the midwife was a nice woman and she could not fault her care but, unfortunately, she looked somewhat similar to a woman who had abused her as a child and she simply could not bear being touched by her. I suggested that she explain this to the midwife, which she did, and the midwife made arrangements for another midwife to take over her care.

Changing your obstetrician

You may get an idea about an obstetrician's views and practices by asking your midwife, childbirth educator, or other women who may have been cared for by him or her, and then make up your own mind. If you decide during your pregnancy that she or he is not for you, then ask your midwife or GP to refer you to another obstetrician. If she or he refuses, you can write to the Chief Executive at your local maternity unit and tell him/her that you no longer wish to be a patient of Mr/Ms X, and would like to be referred to another obstetrician, or to receive midwifery care only. If you decide on midwifery care only, and you need obstetric care later, this will be provided. A midwife has a duty to call for obstetric assistance should she at any time feel there is a need for medical attention, and the doctors have an obligation to respond.

Changing your health visitor

If you wish to change your health visitor, you can either inform the health visitor concerned that you would prefer to be seen by a colleague or you can inform the Head of the GP practice or children's centre and ask for another one to be appointed. Or you can write to the child health clinic, depending upon where the health visitor is based, and ask them to make alternative arrangements.

To summarise, you may change your HP at any time, and if a health professional claims that there is no-one else available you can insist that the Director/Head of Midwifery is called. She has the responsibility to find another HP to attend you. You can be pleasant but assertive. You can also withdraw from care at any time.

A professional's right of access to your home

As mentioned previously, a health visitor has no legal right of access to your home without your consent. Neither do midwives, doctors or social workers, unless they have a Court Order. If you do not wish to see a midwife or health visitor after your baby is born, you might consider taking your baby to a friendly GP so that she or he has been seen, and the HPs cannot then claim that your baby is at risk simply because they have not seen him or her.

Sometimes completely denying access to a newborn baby can lead a health professional to worry that the baby is at risk, and to call, or threaten to call, the police or social services. The police have a right of entry if they think someone may be harmed, but these discussions should always be approached with compassion and care, and fully explained to you by the professionals involved. It is unacceptable for threats to be made simply to gain your compliance.

Am I Allowed: 4th Edition

Chapter 3

Planning Ahead: The Kind of Birth You Want

This chapter discusses the kind of birth you want and the issues surrounding the birth options that are available. This is not about persuading all women to have a particular kind of birth. What is important is that you get support for your decisions and feel safe and understood, wherever and however you decide to give birth. This might be, for example, having a normal birth with midwives or having a planned caesarean with an obstetrician.

A normal birth

"*The infant is born spontaneously in the vertex* [head down] *position between 37 and 42 completed weeks of pregnancy.*" (WHO 1996) Most women hope for and plan to have a normal birth, but in high income countries, the medicalisation of birth has greatly reduced the likelihood of a woman having a normal, straightforward, birth.

There is a wealth of robust evidence showing that the majority of women can birth their babies normally when they are fully informed, have confidence in their ability to give birth, are with people they trust, in surroundings that are quiet, and where they feel safe and are disturbed as little as possible. Becky Reed's book, *Birth in Focus* (2016), shows that good midwifery support enables more women to give birth straightforwardly, but also that any birth, straightforward or not, can be a positive experience when you are well supported. Perhaps every pregnant woman should be given a copy of this book once she knows she is having a baby.

If you want the best chance of being listened to and having your decisions respected, it is worth having some basic knowledge about how birth often unfolds in hospital, what interventions are suggested, what alternatives you might have, and how normal birth is commonly defined. For example, what is often called a normal birth might include any or all of the following: manually breaking the waters (Artificial Rupture of

Membranes – ARM); induction or acceleration of labour; continuous electronic fetal heart monitoring; epidural anaesthesia; episiotomy; and using drugs and certain manoeuvres for the birth of the placenta (a managed third stage). All of these procedures alter the progression of a normal birth, and if a woman has had any of the above then her birth could more accurately be described as an obstetric delivery.

As long ago as 2001, a retrospective review (Downe et al 2001) of women's case notes in five hospitals in the northeast of England found that only 1 in 6 first time mothers, and only 1 in 3 women expecting subsequent babies, actually had a normal birth. Two years later, the Royal College of Midwives launched its *Normal Birth Campaign* to encourage and enable midwives to assist more women to give birth normally.

A survey of seven obstetric units in England (Downe and Finlayson 2016) recorded normal birth rates of 65.5% ranging from 76.5% to 55.6% between those hospitals. Close examination of the data revealed that many of the *normal* births included some form of intervention, reducing the rates to 14.9% for women expecting their first baby and 23.4% for those expecting subsequent babies.

More recently, the NHS Digital (2019) statistics reveal high levels of interventions and that the number of women birthing normally has been further reduced.

Because the official definition of normal birth can include a range of potentially painful interventions, it is not uncommon for some women to believe that their birth, which did include a number of painful interventions, was *normal*. They are left believing that having a normal birth is a dreadful experience and that next time they will opt for an early epidural or caesarean surgery.

Clearly, having a normal birth is not like ordering a pound of flour from the supermarket, where what you order is what you get. To have the best chance of giving birth normally, you need to be well informed and, ideally, able to develop a trusting and equal partnership with your midwife during your pregnancy, in order to develop the confidence that you can labour and birth your baby without unnecessary interventions.

It is that belief and confidence, as well as a realistic picture of what to expect, and a calm environment, that support the flow of birth hormones and enable you to cope with labour without the need for an epidural or other pharmacological drugs. In many areas, HPs strive to provide these calm, homely environments in hospitals, midwifery units, and by supporting home births. However, these conditions are not always easy to create in our current industrialised model of obstetric services, where the midwives and doctors are often overworked and highly stressed (Hunter et al 2018), and where the focus is often on staffing the hospital and getting women through labour as efficiently as possible, rather than supporting you to birth in your own time and way.

It is worth asking your local hospital, Trust or Health Board for the statistics on their intervention rates. You have a right to know what they are before deciding where to give birth. Alternatively, ask your Community Health Council (Wales), Maternity Voices Partnership (England), Patient Advice & Support Service (Scotland) or Patient and Client Council (N Ireland) to obtain these statistics for you.

"Overdue" babies

The medicalisation of birth has resulted in a focus on the baby's *due date*, based on a statistical average length of pregnancy. Rather than estimating that the baby will be due, for example, *in early August,* women are given a specific date, despite *term* being considered to be between 37 and 42 weeks or *"around 40 weeks"* (Middleton et al 2020).

"Only 5% of births occurred on the estimated date of birth, regardless of the dating method or timing of the dating." (Khambalia et al 2013).

"I knew exactly when I conceived as my husband was in the army and he was home for a weekend." This woman repeatedly refused various interventions and, after weeks of arguing, her baby arrived on the date she forecast.

Furthermore, the length of pregnancy can vary by almost three weeks before and past the standard 40 weeks' calculation (Jukic et al 2013). Midwives and women have noticed that longer pregnancies often run in families, so it is useful to find out how long your mother's, sister's, or aunt's pregnancies lasted – excluding those pregnancies where labour has been induced.

"Prolonged gestation may increase risks for babies, including a greater risk of death (before or shortly after birth). However, inducing labour may also have risks for mothers and their babies, especially if the woman's cervix is not ready to go into labour. Current tests cannot predict the risks for babies or their mother, as such, and many hospitals have policies for how long pregnancies should be allowed to continue." (Middleton et al 2020).

It is not uncommon for women to be told that if they go beyond their *due date* their baby could die, without giving them any information about the actual risks. A study by Cotzias (1999) revealed the risks around term:

Risk of unexplained stillbirth by gestation

At 35 weeks it is	1 in 500
36	1 in 556
37	1 in 645
38	1 in 730
39	1 in 840
40	1 in 926
41	1 in 826
42	1 in 769
43	1 in 633

Cotzias (1999)

Recent research into induction of labour has questioned the value of recommending induction at 41 weeks and three days rather than 42 weeks, pointing out the lack of benefit and the increased risks (Rydahl et al 2019).

Induction of labour has become such a common intervention, now affecting a third of women in the UK, that you may want to look at the risks and benefits in more detail on page 74. You have a right to refuse an induction and await developments if that is what you decide to do.

Medically advised caesarean surgery

"Caesareans are associated with short and long term risk which can extend many years beyond the current delivery and affect the health of the woman, her child, and future pregnancies." (WHO 2015a)

I have, throughout this book, referred mainly to caesarean surgery and not caesarean sections. This is because a caesarean is major surgery and to call it a *section* diminishes its seriousness.

In our present climate caesarean surgery has become normalised. For women and babies who need this potentially life-saving intervention, it is safer than it has ever been in high income countries. It has, however, become clear that when overused, the potential harms outweigh the potential benefits (Sandall 2018).

The caesarean rate for England, in March 2020, had risen to 29%, almost 1 in 3 births, (NHS Digital, 2020); 34.5% in Scotland (Public Health Scotland, 2020); 28% in Wales (Welsh Government, 2018-19); and around 33% in N Ireland (2017-18).

In 2015 the World Health Organisation (WHO) issued a statement that *"caesarean section rates higher than 10% were not associated with reductions in rates of maternal and newborn mortality."* (WHO 2015b).

In some areas, practitioners spend time with women with apparently no medical conditions who request caesarean surgery, to find out why they want this, and to make sure that they are well informed about the potential immediate and longer term risks and benefits to them and their babies, and to explore alternatives if this is what they want.

Unfortunately, it is also the case that some professionals and others who advise elective caesarean surgery dismiss the potential adverse effects as minor. Some women who feel pushed into accepting a caesarean often regret it, and say that they were unaware of the long term implications. The following is an extract from *Informed Choice in Maternity Care* (Ed. Kirkham 2014) and is a quotation from a consultant obstetrician looking back on when she had her first baby as a senior registrar:

"At the time I'd been very much the good little girl. I took the advice of the senior consultant and I've lived to regret it. I simply hadn't anticipated that the decision [to have an elective CS] *would mean so much to me. I suffered with postnatal depression after the birth and eventually I went back to that consultant and told him that the decision had been wrong for me. The next baby I had with a midwife I knew and trusted. It has changed me. It really matters to me that women are helped to make decisions which are right for them, not for the medical profession. I get very angry when I hear women say things like 'Oh well it doesn't matter, as long as the baby is all right.' because I know from my own experience that it matters very much. Sometimes long after the birth it's still mattering."* (Stapleton 2004*).*

Most planned caesareans are carried out because women have been advised that surgery is the safest way for their baby to be born. In order to make that decision you should be given information about the potential risks and benefits of the surgery for you and your baby.

The World Health Organisation (WHO) has become so concerned about unnecessarily high levels of caesarean surgery and their adverse effects that their guidance recommends *"mandatory second opinions for caesarean section indication."* (WHO 2018).

If you are told that you need a caesarean you have a right to ask for a second opinion, and it remains your decision whether or not you accept the caesarean, or continue to plan a vaginal birth

Reasons for planning caesarean surgery

Very few women prefer caesarean surgery without a medical indication. Women who apparently *choose* a caesarean often do so for reasons such as:
- They have been persuaded that this is the best choice.
- They have had a previous caesarean.
- They have had a previous traumatic birth.
- They have experienced previous sexual, psychological or physical abuse.
- They fear pain.
- They fear birth.
- They have watched programmes like *One Born Every Minute*.
- They have listened to their friends' or neighbours' traumatic experiences.

If you want an elective caesarean you can explain your reasons for this and arrangements can usually be made for this to happen. Although you have a right to decline surgery, an obstetrician cannot be forced to undertake surgery if she or he thinks it is unnecessary. If, after a discussion, your obstetrician is not supportive, she or he is obliged to refer you for a second opinion. You can also ask for a second opinion, change your obstetrician or hospital, and contact local or national groups for support with your decision (see Resources, Organisations).

If you decide that a caesarean is the best option for you and your baby you can still make decisions about your birth. If all is well, these can include the date of the surgery; the type of anaesthetic (unless there is a very good reason to have a general anaesthetic, spinal anaesthetic is usually considered safer, as well as allowing you to be awake when your baby is born); who will be with you for the birth; whether or not a screen is used; what music is played; whose voice your baby hears first; having immediate skin to skin contact with your baby; having support for early breastfeeding; having your baby wrapped in your own soft towels; ensuring delayed cord clamping occurs; and whether or not you want to keep your placenta. These things are not always routinely available everywhere, but can often be negotiated.

Vaginal birth after caesarean (VBAC)

Many women who have had previous caesarean surgery wish to have a vaginal birth the next time. Sometimes, women are frightened by accounts of uterine rupture and babies dying and, as a result, their confidence in their own bodies in having a VBAC is undermined. The absolute risk of adverse outcomes for VBAC women and babies is small (Fitzpatrick, 2019). Whichever kind of birth you choose *"There was no strong evidence to suggest a difference in outcomes for the baby between a vaginal birth or a repeat caesarean section"* (NICE 2019).

The reported success rates of planned VBAC vary depending on a woman's individual circumstances and between hospitals, regions and countries, but in England, Scotland and Wales the success rate was 60.4% (NMPA 2017). It is worth asking your local unit for their VBAC rates before making a booking. Numbers were small, but women birthing at home were more likely to have a successful VBAC than those giving birth in an obstetric unit. The risk of an adverse outcome was similar in both settings – 2-3% (Rowe 2015).

In other research *"1.8% of those women attempting a vaginal birth and 0.8% of those having a planned caesarean experienced serious maternal complications."* [such as womb rupture, bleeding or infection] (Fitzpatrick et al 2019).

The RCOG, however, stated that: *"Women should be informed that planned VBAC is associated with an approximately 1 in 200 (0.5%) risk of uterine rupture."* (RCOG 2015a). In other words, a woman has a 99.5% chance of not experiencing this complication, and a woman's risk of dying is very small.

"There is a consensus from the National Institute for Health and Care Excellence [NICE], Royal College of Obstetricians and Gynaecologists [RCOG], American College of Obstetricians and Gynecologists [ACOG]/ National Institutes of Health [NIH] that planned VBAC is a clinically safe choice for the majority of women with a single previous lower segment caesarean delivery." (RCOG 2015a)

For those women who have a planned repeat caesarean, the risk of dying is 13-42 per 100,000, compared with 4-16 per 100,000 for those women who planned a VBAC (RCOG 2015a).

You have the right to have a VBAC in hospital or at home, but the admission criteria for many midwifery units exclude women wanting a VBAC. Some women have successfully negotiated VBACs in these units with the support of a Consultant Midwife, or other senior midwives, and in some areas there are dedicated VBAC clinics run by midwives to support women planning VBACs.

Some women planning a VBAC have been refused access to a midwifery unit, but when they informed the staff that they would have a home birth instead, they found that they were accepted into the midwifery unit after all.

There are supportive groups for mothers in the UK who want either a VBAC or Home Birth After Caesarean (HBAC) (see Resources, Organisations).

Consent forms

The most common consent form a woman will be asked to sign will be for caesarean surgery. If there is an increased risk of hysterectomy, such as with placenta praevia, this is usually explicitly discussed and written on the consent form.

Many consent forms state: *"I consent to such further or alternative operative measures as may be found to be necessary during the course of the procedure and to the administration of a general, local or other anaesthetic for any of these purposes."*

You have the right to sign or delete this section and make it clear that you consent only to the surgery in question and not any other procedure that might arise, unless there is a dire emergency.

Occasionally, women have reported that they felt pressured into signing a consent form. Any woman who feels under pressure to sign a consent form can sign the form adding a note stating that she has done so under duress. Furthermore, if having given your consent you later decide otherwise, you can inform the staff, in writing or verbally, that you withdraw your consent as you have decided otherwise.

A water birth

Increasing numbers of women are choosing to labour and give birth in water, either at home, in a midwifery unit, or in hospital.

There is now a considerable body of research showing that birthing in water is a safe option and should be available to any woman who wants it; this includes during the Covid-19 pandemic (Burns et al 2020).

Evidence suggests that immersion in deep warm water can be effective in reducing the need for drugs for pain relief (Liu et al 2014). Some studies showed that it can reduce:
- the length of labour (Garland 2017, Camargo et al 2018);
- interventions (Burns et al 2012, Lukasse et al 2014);
- transfer rates from community settings (Lukasse et al 2014);
- episiotomies (Henderson et al 2014);
- urinary stress incontinence (Liu et al 2014).

Giving birth in water can also shorten the length of labour and women have a lower risk of serious tears (Ulfsdottir 2017).

For women with Group B Strep (GBS), the results of a study showed that giving birth in water protected babies from GBS infections because *"there might be a wash out effect which protects the children during delivery."* (Zanetti-Dallenbach et al 2006). Sara Wickham's book *Group B Strep Explained* (2019) is an excellent source of further information.

The Cochrane Review on water labour and birth (Cluett et al 2018) states that: *"There is no evidence of increased adverse effects to the fetus/neonate or woman from labouring or giving birth in water. Available evidence is limited by clinical variability and heterogeneity across trials, and no trial has been conducted in a midwifery-led setting"* also adding that labouring in water appears to reduce the need for an epidural.

*what every woman should know **before** she gives birth*

One advantage of using a birth pool is that if it does not work for you, you can, if you want to, leave the pool and have pain relieving drugs or an epidural, whereas other forms of pain relief don't leave you with the option to change your mind so easily.

As early as 1992, the Government Report on maternity services recommended the option of a birthing pool (Winterton Report, Dept Health 1992). The majority of hospitals have one or more pools on the labour ward, and some are happy for you to bring in a portable lined pool. Most Birth Centres and midwifery led units have several pools or even pools in every room. If you are planning a home birth you can borrow, hire or buy your own pool.

All midwives are trained to attend women who labour and birth in water, thus, in any unit offering a pool for pain relief in labour, <u>every</u> midwife in the unit should be competent to look after women giving birth in water. In the UK, the use of birth pools has greatly increased and many midwives are enthusiastic about its benefits. However, women may be told, for example, that:

"*There is no-one available who has experience of a water birth.'*
"*There is someone in the pool."*
"*The pool has not yet been cleaned."*

A woman having a home birth was recently asked by her midwife if she had a concrete floor *"because it is important that the floor is concrete in case we have to cut the pool to get you out of the pool!"* This is not a requirement and I have never heard of pools being cut in order to get women out of them.

Sometimes there is a genuine problem in a hospital, with the plumbing or water supply for example, in which case you can reconsider your options about where to give birth.

In some units, women are told that they cannot use the pool because their baby requires continuous electronic fetal monitoring (EFM). In many other units, however, there is wireless fetal monitoring equipment that you can use in water, and you may decide not to agree to EFM.

Finding so many obstacles in their path some women give up what seems to be an unequal struggle and abandon all thoughts of using water, others decide to birth at home where they can be sure of using a birth pool if and when they want. If this happens to you, you could contact your Consultant Midwife or other senior midwives for support.

Labouring and giving birth in water does not appeal to everyone and sometimes, having got into the pool, you may decide that you want to get out before the birth.

In some hospitals you might be asked to get out of the pool for a variety of reasons. To be made to leave the pool if you do not want to do so can result in a sudden increase in pain and stress. You should always be told the reasons for any recommendation.

Some HPs ask women to get out of the pool to birth the placenta on the grounds of a theoretical risk of water embolism, where water might enter the woman's blood stream. There is no evidence to suggest that any woman who has given birth to the placenta in water has ever suffered a water embolism. You have the right to refuse to get out of the water in these or any other circumstances, though you might want to follow the midwife's advice to leave the pool if, for example, your labour is slowing down, you are bleeding too heavily, or have some other complication.

During your pregnancy you can ask how often the pools are used, and how many women labour in water, or actually give birth in water, which should give you a good idea of how enthusiastic the midwives are about this effective form of pain relief. If you find that there is a reluctance to support labour and birth in water, you might suggest to the staff that they obtain a copy of Dianne Garland's book *Revisiting Waterbirth: An attitude to care* (2017).

Heated water pools

Following a report of a baby who contracted Legionnaires' disease from a pre-heated pool, many hospitals withdrew their water birth service.

The incident provoked Professor Nick Phin, Public Health England's (PHE) head of Legionnaires' disease, to issue a statement (2017):

"This is an extremely unusual situation, which we are taking very seriously. As a precaution, we advise that heated birthing pools, filled in advance of labour and where the temperature is then maintained by use of a heater and pump, are not used in the home setting, while we investigate further and until definitive advice on disinfection and safety is available.

We do not have concerns about purchased or hired pools that are filled from domestic hot water supplies at the onset of labour, provided that any pumps are used solely for pool emptying."

Most hospital water pools do not have a built-in heater system. Instead the water is cooled or heated by water directly from the taps.

What type of pool you choose to use at home is your decision.

Freebirthing

If a baby is born without a midwife in attendance because the baby arrived too quickly for a woman to get to her planned place of birth, or before a midwife arrived, this will be recorded as a BBA (Born Before Arrival) or unattended home birth. Some women decide not to call a midwife because they have been unable to negotiate the kind of care they want, and decide that they have no alternative but to birth alone. This should more accurately be described as *Abandoned Birth*, as those women feel abandoned by the local maternity services.

A small number of women feel that they will birth more safely and easily if they do so without the presence of a midwife. The term *Freebirthing* has been used to describe this decision. The numbers are very small and include healthy women and babies as well as women and babies with potential complications. There is very little research on the safety of freebirthing and it is difficult to draw any conclusions.

In some areas women have been reported to social services on the wrongful grounds that they have put their babies at risk by choosing to freebirth, despite having the right not to call a midwife. *"Women are not obliged to accept any medical or midwifery care or treatment during childbirth and cannot be compelled to accept care unless they lack mental capacity to make decisions for themselves."* (Birthrights 2017a).

A woman herself cannot be prosecuted for birthing her own baby. There is no offence in law. If anyone tells you there is, they are misinformed, ignorant, or lying. A woman has a right to have whomever she wishes at the birth, including husband, partner, friend, relative or doula.

An unqualified person who claims or pretends to be a midwife and who assists a woman's birth could be prosecuted and fined a maximum of £5000. Under the Nursing and Midwifery Order 2001 it is an offence for anyone who is not a registered midwife or doctor to *"attend a woman in childbirth"*. Having your husband, partner, doula, or anyone else of your choice present does not qualify as *offence*. Nor does it mean that emergency help cannot be given by a husband, partner, taxi driver, shopkeeper or paramedic, if needed.

If you have chosen to freebirth, or have had an *abandoned birth*, and have been threatened with social services, you can take the name and, if she is a midwife or health visitor, the PIN number, and the full name of any doctor involved, and report them to the Nursing and Midwifery Council or the General Medical Council. Local or national groups can also be contacted for support (see Resources, Organisations).

Chapter 4
Planning Ahead: Place of Birth

Where you give birth is your decision

*"Where you have your baby **is your choice**, and you should always be supported in this choice."* (NICE 2017)

The right of a woman to choose where to give birth is enshrined in English, Welsh, Scottish and Northern Irish policies, and European (EU) law.

Your choice of where to give birth can have a significant influence on the progress of your labour, your future health and that of your baby.

It often takes women time to inform themselves and decide where it feels right to give birth. Ideally, the decision should be made or revisited in late pregnancy or early labour. In some areas, women are given balanced information about all their options for place of birth and can discuss this again anytime during their pregnancies. In others, women are booked to have their baby in hospital early in pregnancy, without being given enough useful information about the options available. For example, you may not be told that home birth is an option, or that there is a FMU in your area. If this happens and you then discover an alternative, possibly in another Trust or Board, or just decide to change your booking, you are entitled to do this, even late on in pregnancy. You do not have to justify or explain your decision. Unless there is a specific reason for choosing a particular place of birth, it is often worth exploring the different options and talking to other women about their experiences before making a final decision.

It is your decision, however, and it is not conditional on the approval of a consultant obstetrician or anyone else.

Options for place of birth

Health practitioners are required to tell you about your options for place of birth, but many women are still told that they will be booked into their local obstetric unit, without any suggestion that there might be other choices.

Not all areas have all the different options for place of birth, but these can include:
- Home birth
- Free-standing Midwifery Unit (FMU)
- Alongside Midwifery Unit (AMU) - a midwifery-led unit within a consultant unit or teaching hospital, sometimes called a Birth Centre or even Home from Home
- Obstetric unit
- Private obstetric unit or wing

If your area does not have an FMU or AMU, your options might be limited to birth at home or in a consultant unit, unless there is a midwifery unit outside your area that you can access.

You can ask to be informed of all your options regarding place of birth in your area, and visit the WHICH? website to see what is available locally (WHICH? 2019).

Informed choice for a hospital birth

If you suggest a home birth you might be informed about the risks, whereas if you plan to go to hospital you will rarely be informed of the risks of hospital birth despite every place of birth having risks and benefits. A printable consent form detailing some of the risks can be found on the Birth Practice and Politics Forum website www.birthpracticeandpolitics.org/post/2019/05/29/informed-consent-for-giving-birth-in-hospital.

Do I have to decide early on where to give birth?

You do not have to make a decision about where to give birth early in your pregnancy or, in fact, at any point until you are in labour. You can take your time. If you are considering a hospital birth, you may wish to visit those units that are within a reasonable distance before you finally decide. It is also worthwhile checking what their Covid-19 policies are as these vary between hospitals.

In the past, many hospitals drew arbitrary *catchment areas* around themselves and might refuse to accept a woman who lived outside the boundary, but some hospitals have become more flexible about these boundaries.

If your area has a choice of maternity units as, for example, in London or other large cities, you should be able to choose to give birth at any of the hospitals or birth centres, but you may need to be registered with the midwives from your local unit for a home birth, or for midwifery care in your home or local GP surgery. This is because each hospital provides maternity community care for a specific geographical area.

If you are not happy with the booking that has been made for you, you can write to the local Director/Head of Midwifery, or Consultant Midwife, clearly stating what you want and asking for their assistance in making the arrangements. If you experience any problems, you can also contact your local or national groups (see Resources, Organisations).

Outcomes for different places of birth

Before deciding on where to have your baby, you might want to consider some of the outcomes for different birth settings for fit, healthy, women and their babies.

A research study in England (Brocklehurst et al 2011) compared the outcomes of over 64,000 fit and healthy women giving birth to their babies by planned place of birth. It showed that very few babies had problems wherever they were born.

For healthy women having their first babies, adverse outcomes per 1000 babies were:

Obstetric unit	5.3
Homebirth	9.3
Free-standing midwifery unit	4.5
Alongside midwifery unit	4.7

Because the number of deaths was too small to make a comparison, all adverse outcomes, for example fractured clavicles, were included.

For women having subsequent babies it was:

Obstetric unit	3.3
Home birth	2.3
Free-standing midwifery unit	2.7
Alongside midwifery unit	2.4

The study also looked at the way these babies were born. Normal births for healthy women per 100 births were:

Obstetric unit	73.8
Home	92.0
Freestanding midwifery unit	90.7
Alongside midwifery unit	85.9

Caesarean Surgery for healthy women per 100 births:

Obstetric unit	11.1
Home	2.1
Freestanding midwifery unit	3.5
Alongside midwifery unit	4.4

Subsequent research findings consistently show good outcomes for out of hospital births, including good outcomes for women having their first babies at home (Hutton et al 2019).

The current recommendation is that:
"Women should be able to make decisions about [...] where they would prefer to give birth, whether this is at home, in a midwifery unit or in an

obstetric unit, after full discussion of the benefits and risks associated with each option." (National Maternity Review 2016).

Having organised where to have your baby you can change your decision at any time, even during labour.

Out of hospital settings

Given the safety of out of hospital settings, advice and guidelines in the UK recommend that healthy women are supported to give birth in these settings. In 2011 for example, the Welsh Assembly Government stated that there should be an *"adequate capacity to enable women to give birth at home, in a birth centre, a midwifery led unit where that is their choice"* (Welsh Assembly Government 2011). The Assembly advised the Trusts that they should make provision for at least 45% of women to give birth outside an obstetric unit.

NICE urges practitioners to:
"Advise low-risk multiparous women that planning to give birth at home or in a midwifery-led unit (freestanding or alongside) is particularly suitable for them because the rate of interventions is lower and the outcome for the baby is no different compared with an obstetric unit." (NICE 2017)

Despite the evidence that birth in out of hospital settings (midwifery units and home) are safe options for fit and healthy women and babies, research results showed that women who wished to birth in an FMU or at home tended to encounter obstacles and negativity (Coxon et al 2017). This goes some way to explaining why the home birth rate in the UK has only reached 2.1% (ONS 2019), though this is variable throughout the UK. For example, one area of Wales has reached 8% whereas for Northern Ireland the figure is 0.04% (NI Statistics and Research Agency 2017), and 1.17% in Scotland (Ross-Davie 2017).

Home births

Research has shown that it is safer for fit and healthy women to give birth at home (Hutton et al 2019), where they have a greater chance of having a normal, physiological birth and rarely use drugs for pain relief. This is not because these women are more courageous, but because a home birth offers the optimum conditions to enable them to relax and focus on birthing their babies.

No farmer would dream of moving their prize cow or horse during labour because they are very aware of how disruptive this can be, and the last thing they want to do is put their precious, and valuable, animal and its baby at risk. Similarly, moving a woman in labour to unfamiliar surroundings, with the stress of the journey, followed by being attended by strangers, disrupts the natural progression of labour.

Your right to a home birth

Under the NHS Acts of 1946 and 1949 there was a legal duty to provide a home birth service. When the health service was reorganised under the 1968 Act, the legal obligations were not clearly stated and, as a result, NHS hospitals now only have a legal duty to provide a *maternity service*. Nevertheless, hospital employees, under Section 6 of the Human Rights Act (1998), are required to respect women's rights as set out in the European Convention on Human Rights, and Article 8 which guarantees the right to respect for private and family life.

The right to a home birth was tested in 2010, when the European Court of Human Rights considered an application brought by a woman who wished to give birth at home with the assistance of a midwife (*Ternovszky v Hungary*, 2010). The Court found Article 8 included the right about where to give birth and stated: *"The right to choice in matters of child delivery includes the legal certainty that the choice is lawful and not subject to sanctions, directly or indirectly."*

Home birth should always be offered regardless of where you live or your service providers' opinions of home birth. Some GPs, obstetricians, and even some midwives, are not supportive of home birth. This may be because they lack knowledge and experience of it, and/or because they are not supported by the hospital to provide a home birth service, and therefore lack confidence and/or resources.

A Mumsnet survey (Roberts 2020) found that *"only 38% said they were given the opportunity to discuss the benefits of giving birth at home"*.

If a doctor or midwife has defined your pregnancy as being *high risk* you are still entitled to midwifery services, and to have your baby at home if you so wish. Some women who have medical conditions or complications feel that they would birth more easily at home, and may wish to have a discussion with the relevant expert to determine what the advantages and risks of this might be. You can ask the doctors to put the reason for recommending a hospital birth in writing. It is important to establish what they see as the risks. If you disagree with their assessment you do not have to battle alone. There are other women and support groups to help you (see Resources, Organisations).

Whatever your local hospital's policy, staffing levels, views, and organisation of maternity services, every woman in the UK has the right to birth at home:

"If a woman wants to birth at home, even if a service is stretched or her pregnancy is complex, the provider needs to put in place the appropriate support for this." (NHS England 2017)

Home birth provision

The home birth service is provided by community midwives and, in some localities, there are dedicated home birth midwifery teams.

In some areas, community midwives do not book women for a specific place of birth. If a woman is healthy and well, they leave the decision about where to give birth until she is in labour. This usually results in more women birthing at home, especially if continuity of carer is offered because, if all is well, women are likely to feel confident and comfortable with their midwives at home. (Homer et al 2017).

Inappropriate reasons for suggesting that a home birth is not possible

While some women report excellent support from midwives and other HPs for their planned home births, other women report being dissuaded from considering or planning a home birth. The following are examples that women have been given over recent years:

"I'm not allowed to give birth upstairs – this is a safety issue and I'm not allowed to question it. They may need to get me rapidly to hospital and our one flight of stairs would impede this – and ambulance men don't like stairs."

Wherever you live, and whatever your home is like, you still have the right to have your baby at home, and in any room.

"My haemoglobin is low – 10.6 (106g/l)."

Most hospitals suggest that a haemoglobin level below 10.0 (100g/l) would be considered to be low. This in itself does not prevent you from choosing to birth at home or in an FMU. You can discuss the potential risks and benefits with a supportive HP.

Women with GBS are told they must have a hospital birth, as they will require intravenous antibiotics in labour (see Sara Wickham's book *Group B Strep Explained* 2019). They can, of course, decline antibiotics. If, however, a woman plans a home birth and wishes to have prophylactic antibiotics at home she should discuss this with her midwife and, if she is concerned, ask her midwife to arrange a discussion with her local Consultant Midwife or Director/Head of Midwifery.

Any of the reasons above could be a cue to ask if the midwife is reluctant to attend a home birth and for speaking with the Director/Head of Midwifery or Consultant Midwife.

What if I am told there are not enough midwives?

Midwifery services are often so stretched that it is not uncommon for women to be told, often at around 36 weeks, that: *"we are short of midwives so if you go into labour at the weekend/between 6pm and 8am/while midwife Smith is on holiday you will have to come into hospital."*

If you are told that you have to go into hospital if a midwife is unavailable for your home birth, you can contact the Director/Head of Midwifery or Consultant Midwife, and ask for the appropriate home birth service to be arranged for you.

If the response is still not supportive, the next step will be to write a letter to the Chief Executive of your local hospital and the Director/Head of Midwifery and send a copy to the Clinical Commissioning Group (the body that commissions local maternity services in England and Northern Ireland), and the Health Boards in Scotland and Wales, along the following lines:

Dear

I have been informed that you have a shortage of midwives and when I call in labour the Maternity Unit may not be able to send one and I shall, therefore, have to come into hospital.

Your service has been aware of my intention to give birth at home since ....(insert date). I have no intention of taking the additional risk of a hospital birth because of your staff shortages, although I am prepared to transfer to hospital should a medical complication arise.

We expect a midwife to attend when called to my labour. Should a midwife not arrive we will consider that I have been abandoned by your hospital. Should any untoward event occur that is related to your failure to respond to my needs and those of my baby, my family will take appropriate action and we shall hold you and the Director/Head of Midwifery personally responsible for this failure.

If you are concerned about the greater risk of contracting Covid-19 in hospital, you can add this to your letter.

What to do if your midwife is not supportive

If your midwife is not enthusiastic, skilled, and supportive, you can ask her how she feels about attending home births, and ask her about her experience. One of the advantages of booking a home birth is that it offers a better chance of getting to know the midwife who will actually attend you in labour and finding out:
- when she last attended a woman giving birth at home;
- how many home births she has attended;
- how many women she has transferred to hospital in labour;
- what emergencies can occur in a home birth, and how she would deal with them to facilitate your and your baby's safety, such as if your baby was unexpectedly in the breech position; and
- what back up she can call on.

If it emerges that she has little experience of home birth, ask her what measures she will put in place to ensure she has a second, more experienced midwife to support her.

If you are still not happy with the midwife allocated to your care, or are concerned about her experience or competence, it is always better to act during your pregnancy rather than leave it until you are in labour, when you are less likely to be able to assert yourself. You can suggest that the midwife finds another colleague to attend you or you can write to the Director/Head of Midwifery or Consultant Midwife at your nearest maternity unit, and ask for another midwife to attend you. Occasionally, this has proved difficult, but if the same midwife arrives at your home you can refuse her admission and request another midwife. You can also inform your Maternity Voices Partnership or other local or national support groups (see Resources, Organisations).

Sometimes, if midwives lack confidence in attending a birth at home, they might find a reason to justify taking you into hospital during labour, such as telling you that that your labour is not progressing quickly enough. You can ask her if there is a problem with your baby and if she says that there is not, and you feel that you are managing, you can suggest that she waits a couple of hours and then review the situation rather than agree to go in immediately.

How to secure midwifery services when you are in labour at home

If you ring for a midwife while in labour and are told that a midwife is not available for you due to staff shortages, you, or your partner, can ask for the answering midwife's name and PIN number. Make a note of these and ask to speak to the on-call manager of the unit, the matron or the Director/Head of Midwifery, even if out of hours, and then state:
I have no intention of putting myself/my partner or my/our baby at risk of travelling in labour to the hospital and exposing us/them to the additional risks of a hospital delivery. If you fail to send a midwife and any untoward event occurs which can be attributed to your failure to provide a midwife you can rest assured that my family will take appropriate action.

One woman commented on her experience:
"I did get my home birth in the end which was perfect and resulted in a beautiful little girl but I had to argue it on the morning I called up in labour. They said they had no one to send and I'd have to go in to the hospital. When I refused they miraculously found me two midwives who arrived about 45 minutes before our baby was born. If I had not felt so confident about it I would have felt pressured to go to hospital and my homebirth wouldn't have happened."

You should not have to battle while in labour but women and partners who stand their ground are often those who achieve their home birth.

Two midwives attending a home birth

In most areas of the UK, the usual practice is for the primary midwife to come to your home when called, assess your progress, and only call a second midwife shortly before your baby is born. Many services insist that two midwives attend a woman birthing at home. Sometimes you may be asked if a student midwife can also come. A second midwife, or student midwife, attending can have a number of advantages:

- The first midwife may not have much experience of a home birth and a second midwife can be a considerable support.

- You might develop a complication or be expecting a breech baby, in which case a second midwife can be invaluable. If you are expecting twins you will usually have three midwives, one for the mother and one for each of the babies. Although rare, particularly if you have had scans, it is possible that an undiagnosed breech presentation or twins could emerge, and every midwife attending a home birth should know how to deal with these situations and will seek appropriate help.
- Although not yet a qualified midwife, a student would benefit from experiencing normal birth at home and may provide additional support.

Some women are happy – indeed delighted – to have two midwives at the birth, others report that they found it intrusive and that it affected the intimate atmosphere of their home birth, and sometimes the midwives spent more time relating to each other than to the labouring woman. If you are uncomfortable with two midwives it is always possible for the second midwife to stay in another room unless she is needed.

You are under no obligation to accept two midwives into your house, or in the room where you are labouring.

While there are some women who feel more confident birthing alone, there are circumstances where a midwife's knowledge and skill can be essential. A few years ago, I was contacted by a couple who asked the midwife to stay outside the room while the woman was inside with a doula. The baby was born and the doula left the room to tell the midwife and the father that the baby had arrived. As soon as the midwife saw the baby she realised that it was in distress. She took immediate action and all was well, but neither the doula nor the father had been aware of the seriousness of the baby's condition.

Home birth after a caesarean (HBAC)

If you plan to give birth vaginally after a caesarean you might be told that you *have to* give birth in hospital. While many women will be happy to plan a hospital birth, you may feel that hospital is not appropriate and decide to stay at home, where there is less chance of unnecessary interventions and you will benefit from having a midwife in attendance all the time, once labour is well established.

You have the right to birth at home, even if you have had previous caesarean surgery, and the hospital has a responsibility to send you a midwife. There are support groups for women planning HBAC (see Resources, Organisations).

Postnatal examination of the baby at home

The current recommendation is that babies have a thorough physical check within 72 hours of the birth (Newborn Infant Physical Examination – NIPE), to detect possible hip, heart, eye, or other problems.

Many midwives are trained to do a neonatal examination of a baby. The midwife has a responsibility to make arrangements for one to be done, but it is not obligatory and you have the right to decline. If your midwife is not able to do this check, and recommends that you attend the hospital instead, you can, if you choose, point out that you are not willing to put yourself, or your baby, at the additional risk of entering a hospital, nor are you willing to leave your home at this time. If they want to carry out the newborn examination then a GP or another midwife can come to your home to do one.

Free-standing Midwifery Unit (FMU)/Birth Centres

These freestanding units are not located on the same site as an obstetric unit and are sometimes referred to as Birth Centres. They are run entirely by midwives and focus on supporting women to birth safely without interventions. They are usually very popular among the women and families who use them and many midwives enjoy working in them.

They tend only to accept *low risk* women, and therefore women who book there are unlikely to need the range of technology available in consultant units. Women who have been labelled *high risk* or have *additional needs* have sometimes been able to negotiate and book into these units, for example, women who plan a Vaginal Birth After Caesarean (VBAC). The guidelines for admission are not set in stone and can be negotiated with the senior midwife at the Birth Centre, the Director/Head of Midwifery or a Consultant Midwife.

At the time of writing, there were 61 FMUs/Birth Centres in England, two in Northern Ireland, 17 in Scotland and 13 in Wales, and, in every region other than Northern Ireland, these numbers have gone down during the last two years (National Maternity and Perinatal Audit 2019) and, of the remainder, many are under constant threat of closure. In the present financial climate it is easier to close these units, despite the fact that Midwifery Units offer fit and healthy women and babies safe care, fewer interventions, and better outcomes.

If you are planning to birth in a freestanding unit you could enquire about whether or not there are any impending/temporary closures and how this may affect you. If this is likely, you can alert national and local support groups (see Resources, Organisations) or write to the Director/Head of Midwifery at the hospital and complain about their failure to provide a service appropriate to your needs.

If you need help during your labour, the midwives will transfer you in plenty of time to a consultant unit. Research has shown that while *"most transfers are not urgent, and emergencies and adverse outcomes are uncommon, but urgent transfer was more likely for nulliparous women [first time mothers]"* (Rowe et al 2013). It is speculated that this could be caused by midwives acting cautiously when the labour is not progressing as anticipated. Many units have found that as the midwives become more skilled and confident at attending normal births the transfer rates reduce. For example, at the Montrose Midwifery Unit in Scotland *"the intrapartum transfer rate fell from 21% in 2002 to 8% in 2005"* (Winters 2006).

Alongside Midwifery Unit (AMU)

These units are situated within or alongside an obstetric unit and may also be called Birth Centres or Home from Home Units. Due to financial and medical concerns, there has been more support from medical staff and management for AMUs than for FMUs, despite the evidence of better outcomes in FMUs.

Because AMUs are in close proximity to an obstetric unit, midwives are often expected to work in both the AMU and the obstetric labour ward. As a result, they do not have as much opportunity for honing their midwifery skills and supporting normal birth as they would have in an FMU or at home, and some AMUs have higher transfer rates than FMUs (Rowe et al 2012).

The difficulty for women is how to determine whether or not an AMU really offers an opportunity to give birth normally, or whether the normal birth rate is similar to the obstetric unit. The BirthPlace Study showed that intervention rates are lower at home than those for comparable healthy women in the AMUs or consultant units (Brocklehurst et al 2011). This may be because these units are under the influence of obstetric practice. You may want to visit your AMU, if you have one locally, and talk to the midwives, and ask for their current intervention and transfer rates. You will get a feel for their philosophy of care during your visit, which can help you to make a decision about the best place for you to give birth.

Consultant Units (OUs)

Consultant, or obstetric, units (OUs) are designed primarily to provide services for women and babies with additional obstetric or medical needs. In the past, all women were booked with a consultant obstetrician, but in recent years this system has changed so that most women can book directly with their local midwife and then be referred to an obstetrician, if necessary. You can request obstetric services through your GP or midwife.

Some women feel safer in an obstetric unit under the care of an obstetrician, especially if they have got to know her or him. For women with obstetric, medical or other conditions these units have the staff and technology to look after them and their babies if it is needed. Many OUs have specialist services for women with diabetes, women having twins or more, women having vaginal breech births and women who plan what is sometimes called a *gentle caesarean section*. This involves, as far as possible, making a planned caesarean section focus on the birth of the baby rather than solely on the surgical operation, by considering who will be present, how they will behave and the physical factors in the room: all of this can potentially be negotiated beforehand. Similarly, within the obstetric unit you might create a safe and comfortable space with your partner/s by using things such as your own food, music or low lighting.

Your community midwife or Consultant Midwife may be able to tell you about the views and practices of individual consultants, as these can vary. It is possible to change consultants if you are unhappy, or ask for a second opinion from another consultant if you feel that you are not being given the right treatment or care options.

Consultant, or obstetric, units vary in size considerably, with between 2,500 and over 10,000 births a year.

Fit and healthy women giving birth in larger OUs generally have higher levels of caesarean surgery and other interventions, and fewer normal births (Downe and Finlayson 2016). If your hospital has not made its outcomes available publicly on its website or via the WHICH? website, then you have a right to contact the Chief Executive, or Medical Director, and ask for the data.

Sometimes you might not be able to give birth in the unit you have chosen because the hospital is full and it would be unsafe to admit more women in labour. In these circumstances, you would be advised to go to the next nearest unit that has space. In 2017 almost half the maternity units in England were closed temporarily, for shorter or longer periods (Ewers 2018).

There are very few private obstetric units, and most are in London. If you choose to book into a private obstetric unit you might wish to know that although they provide a very good hotel service, most private consultant units have high caesarean and intervention rates and, unlike NHS hospitals, they do not have the facilities to deal with serious obstetric emergencies and in rare circumstances women may be transferred to an NHS hospital if such care is needed.

Am I Allowed: 4th Edition

Chapter 5
Antenatal Services

"The case for change in maternity services is compelling and widely accepted. All women deserve to receive care which is safe, both physically and emotionally. This means receiving the right care from the right person at the right time in the right setting, according to the woman's needs." (Northern Ireland 2017). The English, Scottish and Welsh governments have made similar statements. (see Resources, Maternity Policies).

Confirming your pregnancy

Home pregnancy kits are obtainable from the chemist, online, or from some supermarkets. These have enabled women to confirm their pregnancies very early, and in privacy, allowing time to think about what they want before consulting anyone.

You may be able to access free pregnancy testing from GPs, NHS walk in health centres and sexual health clinics or, if you don't want to use a test, you can ask your local midwives to confirm your pregnancy, but during the pandemic all arrangements need to be checked.

Organising antenatal care

Once you know you are pregnant, you can book an appointment directly with your community midwife. If you are unsure about how to contact a midwife or the GP's surgery, the Children's Centre or local childbirth organisations/charities will be able to put you in touch. If you have internet access you can also check online.

You can check arrangements for antenatal care during the pandemic through your midwife or on your local hospital's website. In some areas, women see the same midwife or two during pregnancy, in others they might see any number of midwives. A number of women still report seeing a different midwife at each appointment. The only women who have a greater chance of continuity of care from one or two midwives are those who have an NHS community based case-load midwifery group in their area, or who book an independent or private midwife, or who see an obstetrician privately.

Some women feel very anxious in early pregnancy and can often feel that they are not getting enough care. If you would like to see a midwife to discuss this, you can phone your local community midwifery office, or if you still are not getting the care you need, you can contact your Director or Head of Midwifery.

If you have a health condition, or possible complications, or want to see an obstetrician, your midwife can refer you to one, whether or not you have any additional needs which mean you need to see a specialist as well. The obstetrician is an expert in complicated pregnancies, but you will continue to have a midwife to provide ongoing care and support.

Frequency of antenatal appointments

The frequency of antenatal appointments in the UK is based on advice from the National Institute for Health and Care Excellence (NICE 2019), which suggests that a healthy woman with an uncomplicated pregnancy should receive up to ten antenatal appointments if she is a first time mother (primiparous or primip) and even if she has had a baby before (a multiparous or multip).

The current recommendations for healthy women are to have a booking appointment, *"between 8 to 12 weeks pregnant, a dating scan at 8-14 weeks and then have a check at 16 weeks, 18 - 20 weeks, 25 weeks (primips only), 28 weeks, 31 weeks (primips only), 34 weeks, 36 weeks, 38 weeks, 40 weeks (primips only), 41 weeks and 42 weeks"* (NHS Health A-Z 2020). For those who have not given birth by 41 weeks a further visit is recommended to discuss induction of labour, or a membrane sweep, but many HPs will want to discuss this at around 40 weeks or earlier. You are entitled to full information about induction and membrane sweeps and can then accept, decline, await events or reconsider later. If you wait, you may be offered further monitoring and you are entitled to accept or refuse that too. Sara Wickham's book *Inducing Labour – Making Informed Decisions* (2018) has a helpful section discussing these options in more depth.

Your midwife should provide you with details about how to contact her for additional appointments should you not feel well, or are worried about your baby, or wish to discuss something in between these routine appointments.

Choosing antenatal classes

NHS antenatal classes are provided by many maternity units. The effectiveness of these classes have yet to be determined (Gagnon and Sandall 2007), though some approaches have been found to reduce stress and anxiety during pregnancy. (Çankaya and Şimşek (2020).

Some NHS hospitals offer hypnobirthing, yoga or mindfulness classes, as well as the traditional antenatal classes, although some are now offering women videos instead, due to a shortage of midwives, pressures within the NHS, and Covid-19 restrictions. You can check local NHS arrangements for antenatal classes during the pandemic, as many initially moved to electronic formats, although some have started in-person sessions again.

Some NHS antenatal classes are run by enthusiastic midwives who provide women and their partners with excellent information based on research and their own wealth of experience. Some women, however, report that there is a shortage of classes or that they tend to prepare women to accept the services the hospital offers.

Women are not always given sufficient information to enable them to make informed decisions about where and how they would like to have their baby, or discuss the pros and cons of an intervention that may be offered during their pregnancy or labour. Some women find that even when they have been given good information, once they get into hospital it can be difficult to act on it.

Am I Allowed: 4th Edition

Many private childbirth educators and charitable organisations provide classes and workshops to prepare parents for the birth of their baby. Content and fees for these vary, but some do offer free or reduced price classes to parents who cannot afford to pay. There are voluntary organisations and charities established to give women support and information about a wide range of maternity issues. The Pregnancy and Parents Centre in Edinburgh is one example (see Resources, Organisations).

You may wish to explore what options are available in your area.

Parents can sign up for NHS antenatal classes and also attend private classes. Many report that they gain different benefits from the various sessions.

Chapter 6
Screening and Diagnostic Tests

There are wide variations in pregnancy care across the UK and elsewhere. Midwives do the best they can to support pregnant women through what can be a challenging, as well as a joyful, time. Overall, however, for the last few decades, more and more of the midwives' time has had to be spent on testing and monitoring, leaving less time to explore a woman's feelings and concerns and provide her with the emotional support she needs.

There are many tests which are offered during pregnancy and new tests are being developed all the time.

You may wish to have some screening tests for a particular reason, or consider whether or not to embark on any screening during your pregnancy. Some women have said that they had not properly thought about the implications of having a test until they were informed that there was a possible problem. Some have said that they wished that they had not had some of the tests, because they felt forced into further decisions they would have preferred to avoid or, when there was an adverse result, some have reported feeling under pressure to abort their baby rather than awaiting events. Other women prefer to have whatever tests are available, as they feel that this will help them prepare to deal with any future problem should it arise. No matter what tests are developed in the future, <u>the decision whether or not to have them is yours</u>.

The tests undertaken in pregnancy can be divided into two types: screening tests and diagnostic tests. The main screening tests are done using ultrasound scans or carried out on blood and urine samples.

A **screening test** can be compared to going through an airport security check. The alarm bells ring suggesting that you might be carrying a weapon, but careful examination reveals that you have left a coin in your pocket. If a screening test suggests that there could be a possible problem, a **diagnostic test** will then be suggested to check whether or not there really is a problem.

No screening or diagnostic test is 100% accurate.

You can find that you end up with a *false negative*, an indication that there is nothing wrong when there is; or a *false positive*, an indication that there is something wrong when there is not.

Identifying a possible problem does not necessarily indicate its severity. Some problems can be very serious, but fortunately these are rare, and many babies with serious problems sadly either die during the pregnancy or shortly afterwards.

It is also possible for a problem to be identified when one does not exist. Anecdotally, one of the most common comments made to women is that the baby is too big, or too small, for dates and, since predicting birth weight either by ultrasound or palpation is known to be inaccurate, this can often cause anxiety needlessly.

In some areas, women are given detailed information appropriate to their individual circumstances, and given time to decide before being offered any antenatal testing. This does not happen universally. If you do not have all the information you need before you decide whether or not to accept specific tests, you can request more.

Questions to ask:
- What is the test for?
- Why are you suggesting it in my case? You might be told *"Oh, this is our policy"*. This does not mean that it will automatically benefit each individual, and just because it is policy you do not have to agree to it.
- What are the chances of an adverse outcome for my baby or for me? For example, is there a chance I could miscarry?
- If the test suggests a poor outcome, what will be the next step/recommendation?
- How many false positive or false negative results are there? You can ask for the national statistics and the hospital's own statistics and compare them.

- Can you show me the study or studies that support the advice or information I have been given?

Some procedures, such as blood pressure and urine testing, are offered at each antenatal appointment, others at specific times or for specific reasons.

For more information see NHS website – Screening tests in pregnancy.

The following are some of the most common procedures and tests currently offered.

Body Mass Index (BMI)

Our society has become obsessed with women's size, and as a result there are implications for women who are even slightly or moderately heavier or lighter than average.

The BMI is a tool that can be used to assess a person's weight compared to their height. If you know your height and weight, you can work out which weight range you're in by using the NHS website calculator (NHS Health 2018).

The BMI weight classification, as defined by the WHO, is outlined as follows:
- If your BMI is less than 18.4, you're underweight for your height.
- If your BMI is between 18.5 and 24.9, you're an ideal weight for your height.
- If your BMI is between 25 and 29.9, you're over the ideal weight for your height.
- If your BMI is between 30 and 39.9, you're classified as obese.
- If your BMI is over 40, you're classified as very obese.

If your BMI is over 25 or under 18.4 then assumptions may be made by HPs without considering, for example, whether or not you are fit and healthy, or whether or not you have a large or small frame.

While women who are very overweight or underweight do have increased risks during pregnancy and labour, they are also more likely to have unnecessary interventions. Having a high or low BMI does not necessarily mean that you will have complications during pregnancy or labour.

In some areas, women with a high BMI are encouraged to see an anaesthetist during their pregnancy and advised to have an epidural during labour in case complications arise. You may wish to consider this option but you equally may wish to be active and mobile in labour, to improve your chances of labour progressing well, and you have the right not to see the anaesthetist or have an epidural during labour.

Blood pressure (BP)

During your pregnancy your midwife will ask to check your BP regularly as this can confirm that it is normal, or give an early indication that there may be a developing problem such as pre-eclampsia – a collection of symptoms which include some or all of the following: high blood pressure; swelling of the feet, ankles, face and hands caused by fluid retention; protein in the urine; headaches and/or visual disturbances; and abdominal pain. This is a serious condition if left untreated, so it is important to alert your midwife should you develop any of these symptoms.

Normal blood pressure during pregnancy ranges from 110/60 to 140/90 and your norm can be anywhere in between. At 140/90 a midwife may check the reading again and discuss further action. She will become concerned should the lower figure rise more than 20 points during your pregnancy. She will discuss with you what further action might be needed, such as a referral to an obstetrician. The guidelines are published in Hypertension in pregnancy: diagnosis and management NICE guideline [NG133], published date: 25 June 2019.

Urine testing

A urine test can show whether or not you have protein, ketones, or sugar in your urine, and measures, for example, the number of white blood cells, or the presence of nitrates, which can indicate the presence of infection. Sugar in your urine could suggest that you may have diabetes, which is a disease caused by your body producing too little insulin. If there is protein in the urine this may simply be caused by the sample having some vaginal secretions in it, or you may have an infection, or it may be a sign of pre-eclampsia or diabetes, and your midwife will suggest further tests, treatments and/or a referral to an obstetrician.

Blood tests

At the first antenatal appointment a woman will be offered several blood tests, which will include some or many of the following:
- your blood group and whether or not your blood group contains the Rhesus factor or any unusual antibodies;
- your haemoglobin level (Hb) – to check if you are anaemic (low in iron);
- if you have syphilis (a sexually transmitted disease that can be passed onto the baby);
- if you have had hepatitis B; or
- if you have the Human Immunodeficiency Virus (HIV) (the test is now routinely offered throughout the UK).

Note: The blood test that examines the iron content in the blood, which, in early pregnancy, should be around 102-130g/l (often written as 10.2-13). As the pregnancy progresses women's blood volume increases so that the haemoglobin content (Hb) in a normal pregnancy appears to drop. A decrease of around 20g/l is expected and beneficial to your baby's growth, and if you are expecting twins there could be a further decrease (see Frye 1997).

If a midwife is suggesting that your Hb is too low (below 100g/l at term, although different areas have different cut-off points), you can ask her if she has checked the mean cell volume (MCV) and/or the ferritin level. This is a better indicator of your iron stores and should be between 80-100g/l.

If both the Hb and MCV are low the midwife may wish to check your blood iron stores (ferritin) before prescribing an increase in iron intake. If the levels are just slightly low the midwife should discuss with you how this might be improved by diet.

One of the reasons that a woman's haemoglobin is measured is because if it is low and she bleeds excessively during or after the birth she could become unwell.

Women who book their care with an independent/private midwife are sometimes told by maternity services that they will have to make arrangements for blood and other tests privately. This is untrue, as women are entitled for these to be carried out on the NHS. If a midwife finds that the GP or hospital are uncooperative, the midwife can contact her Consultant Midwife or Director/Head of Midwifery who will be able to make the necessary arrangements.

Screening tests for rare conditions

Screening tests are available to identify your baby's chance of developing a number of rare conditions, and Down's Syndrome (Trisomy 21) is one example. The Gov.uk website *"Screening tests for you and your baby"* has further information.

Diagnostic tests

If the screening tests suggest that your baby has a higher risk of having a specific rare condition you will be offered an amniocentesis or possibly chorionic villus sampling. A newer kind of screening test, Non-Invasive Prenatal Testing (NIPT) may be available to you within the NHS, during the first trimester, depending on where you live. This is a blood test taken from the mother that uses cutting edge DNA technology to evaluate whether a baby has a high chance of a certain chromosomal condition. The GOV.UK website *"Fetal anomaly screening: CVS and amniocentesis information for parents"* has further information.

Domestic abuse

Domestic abuse is common, and estimated to affect approximately one in four women at some point in their lives. Because domestic abuse commonly starts or escalates during pregnancy, it is now routine to ask screening questions which allow those experiencing abuse to get help and support. Just because your HP asks the questions, it does not mean that they think you are at risk, it is because it is not always easy to spot the signs and it is easier to ask for help if someone asks you directly than if they expect you to say something. Domestic abuse is more than physical violence. It includes verbal abuse, isolating or controlling behaviour, stalking, intimidation, economic control and sexual abuse, and often does not get better over time but, more commonly, gets worse, particularly during pregnancy. Domestic abuse can also have a significant impact on children, so getting help is important for the whole family. If you are experiencing abuse from someone in your family, someone you live with or a former partner, it is domestic abuse and help is available. If you do not feel comfortable talking to your HP there are other sources of help and support. Women's Aid (www.womensaid.org.uk) and Refuge (www.refuge.org.uk) have explanations, self-help and legal information, and resources for helping those who may be experiencing abuse and for those who are concerned for others.

Ultrasound

This section is longer and more detailed than other ones. There are two reasons for this. First, both Jean Robinson and I have been concerned for several decades that the screening for ultrasound was brought in, and has become widely used, before evidence of possible long-term effects was available (Beech and Robinson 1994) but, as explained below, it is now difficult to run randomised controlled trials. The second reason is that although there are some studies, they are not widely available and accessed and so women are not able to make properly informed decisions. So, at the risk of making this book a little 'lopsided' I have included information not widely available elsewhere.

Nearly all women in the UK and many other countries will be offered routine scans during their pregnancies. The number of scans varies from country to country. In most areas of the UK you will be offered an early scan from 8 weeks to 14 weeks to confirm your pregnancy and estimate when your baby is due, and a further scan between 18 and 21 weeks to check whether or not your baby has any specific problems, and to establish the position of the placenta. If you have potential or existing medical or obstetric complications you will be offered more regular scans. Very early trans-vaginal and late scans are now increasingly common but you can accept or decline any ultrasound examinations.

Many ultrasound departments have stopped companions and children attending during the Covid-19 crisis. You can check with your midwife or the hospital to find out what restrictions are in place or look at your local maternity unit's website. Many departments, however, have now lifted the restriction on companions.

Scans have been used in maternity care for over 60 years. The Royal College of Obstetricians and Gynaecologists has consistently maintained that ultrasound is safe when used for clinical reasons. It can be a valuable tool when used to identify a problem, for example, to diagnose an ectopic pregnancy where the fertilised egg has developed in a woman's uterine tube and can be life threatening if undetected.

There have, however, been no human studies designed to check long-term safety, by which I mean at least 10 to 20 years hence, despite repeated requests to do so (Beech 2014). As long ago as 1976 it was claimed that as *"ultrasound techniques have become so widespread that a controlled trial along the lines originally proposed would no longer be ethically possible."* (Medical Research Council 1976).

Not only is ultrasound widely used, but the machines are now far more powerful than those that were developed initially and used in subsequent animal studies.

While almost every unborn child in the UK is exposed to increasingly more powerful ultrasound, its long-term effects remain unevaluated.

Doppler devices

Doppler ultrasound, a more powerful form of ultrasound, is used to study blood flow in the unborn baby, uterus and the placenta.

The Cochrane Systematic Review concludes that *"Existing evidence does not provide conclusive evidence that the use of routine umbilical artery Doppler ultrasound, or combination of umbilical and uterine artery Doppler ultrasound in low-risk or unselected populations benefits either mother or baby."* (Alfirevic et al 2015**).**

Hand-held Doppler devices are also used to listen to the baby's heartbeat, and some parents have bought them to listen to the baby's heartbeat in the comfort of their own homes, perhaps unaware that these Doppler devices emit a powerful version of ultrasound, which is at least ten times more powerful than those used earlier, and new machines are being developed all the time. If you prefer not to use ultrasound, you can ask your midwife to use a pinard or fetal stethoscope.

Keepsake videos

Women are often encouraged to have extra ultrasound in order to have a picture or video of their baby taken by commercial companies, who advertise *Keepsake Videos* of babies in the womb, accompanied with claims that ultrasound is *safe*. The medical profession has warned that *Keepsake Videos* are only safe in professional hands, and that *"souvenir [keepsake] ultrasound is not recommended since the benefits cannot outweigh any potential risks."* (RCOG 2015b). Scan photos are sometimes made available as part of NHS screening.

Ultrasound for low-lying placenta

If you have an anomaly scan at 18-21 weeks, you may be told that you have a low-lying placenta. Grade I indicates a placenta that is farthest away from the cervix and Grade IV refers to a placenta that entirely covers the cervix. At the end of pregnancy, only a few placentas will cover or partially cover the cervix (placenta praevia). In most cases, due to the way your uterus expands, your placenta moves out of the way as the pregnancy develops.

No recent research has been carried out, but a large randomised controlled trial (Saari-Kemppainen et al 1990) of 9,310 pregnant women diagnosed four women with Grade IV placenta praevia, and four other women who did not have ultrasound also had placenta praevia at term. All eight women had caesarean surgery and there was no difference in the health of their babies.

There is no evidence that early detection of a low-lying placenta by ultrasound improves the outcome for mother and baby. Although there have been further studies, (such as Bronsteen 2009) this evidence is still valid as further studies have not refuted these findings.

Ultrasound for estimating baby's weight

It is not uncommon for a woman to be told during pregnancy that her baby might be too small or too large. Interestingly, a study comparing clinicians' estimates of babies' weight, by ultrasound, with the women's estimates of their baby's weight, found that the most accurate assessments were made by women, at term, who had already had a baby (Ashrafganjooei et al 2010).

While ultrasound scans can provide invaluable information that is unavailable through other means, the RCOG cautions that:
"While serial ultrasound screening has moderate predictive value in high-risk women, it has limited accuracy to predict a SGA [Small for Gestational Age] *baby or adverse neonatal outcomes in women without significant risk factors and is therefore not recommended in this population."* (RCOG 2013). See NICE guidelines for more information.

Research studies

The opportunity to carry out large, randomised controlled trials, with long-term follow up, in the early stages of ultrasound development, was rejected by the Medical Research Council (1985). Numerous animal studies, however, were carried out to investigate possible adverse effects. Animal studies provide limited knowledge for humans, and cannot be assumed to apply to humans, but they can provide pointers. These studies have identified behavioural changes in animals (Tarantal et al 1993 and McClintic et al 2013); and changes in neural migration (Ang et al 2006). As early as 1993 Tarantal's study showed that monkey babies exposed to ultrasound in the womb behaved differently to those who were not exposed. Baby monkeys exposed to ultrasound sat or lay around the bottom of the cage, whereas the control monkeys were up to the usual monkey tricks.

Human brain development

Despite a lack of research into ultrasound's possible effects on human babies, concern has been expressed about ultrasound's effect on a baby's developing brain (Bello and Ekele 2012).

Jim West, an American environmental researcher, published a bibliography of fifty Chinese ultrasound research papers (West 2015 and West 2017). Following the one child policy in China, and with women's consent, the Chinese researchers were able to examine the brains of over two and a half thousand aborted babies, who had been exposed to ultrasound in utero. The researchers concluded that ultrasound caused significant changes in the babies' brain structures and, as a result of their findings, they recommended that:
- Ultrasound should only be used for specific medical indications.
- If used, clinicians should strictly adhere to the smallest dose required to obtain the necessary diagnostic information in as short a time as possible.
- Keepsake videos for entertainment should be banned.

- Where possible, ultrasound in the first trimester [before 12 weeks] should be avoided, and during the second or third trimester its use limited to three to five minutes.

Until Jim West's bibliography of Chinese ultrasound research papers there had not been sufficiently rigorous research to determine ultrasound's safety. The Chinese studies raise concerns that should not be dismissed, and clinicians should be cautious and so should we.

Accepting or declining ultrasound examinations

Some women find pregnancy scans reassuring and would prefer more scans than they are offered. Some women say that they feel they have to agree to whatever ultrasound examinations are recommended. It is important to understand that while an ultrasound examination might provide useful information for individual women and babies:
- its safety for unborn babies remains neither proven nor disproven;
- the information gained may make no difference to the course of your pregnancy or outcome;
- it may be suggested for research purposes, but unnecessary for your care;
- it may not be accurate;
- it may cause on-going anxiety.

Your HP should explain why a scan is being recommended and what the benefits and risks are thought to be. If a problem is suspected what action can be taken? In the majority of instances there is little that can be done, other than to await the arrival of your baby, or terminate your pregnancy. If the diagnosis is not accurate, you may have many months of unnecessary anxiety. As with any treatment, you can ask questions or ask for a second opinion, and you have every right to accept or decline an ultrasound examination.

Chapter 7
Decision Making in Late Pregnancy, Labour, and Birth

Because of hormonal changes, the process of labour is very sensitive to a woman's emotions. If you are disturbed, anxious, or worried, your labour can become painful and may not progress straightforwardly and interventions may be offered. This is because the woman's production of oxytocin, which is essential for labour, and an essential safety feature to avoid birth in dangerous situations, is inhibited by stress hormones.

When women are well supported, in an environment where they feel safe, comfortable and undisturbed, labour usually goes well, thus any procedures, interventions, examinations, and questions are best kept to a minimum.

This chapter covers some of the more common procedures, examinations and interventions that may be offered to you during pregnancy, labour, birth and immediately after birth. You may want to find out about them, what they involve and the potential benefits and risks, so that you can discuss them and make a decision about whether to accept or decline.

Stretch and sweep

In late pregnancy, prior to going into labour, you may well be offered a *stretch and sweep* of your membranes. This is an intervention often used to try and start labour before your body naturally goes into labour. It does not always work and it can be painful. The use of this intervention varies across the UK. The authors of the Cochrane Review (Finucane et al 2020) concluded that:
"Membrane sweeping may be effective in achieving a spontaneous onset of labour, but the evidence for this was of low certainty. When

compared to expectant management, it potentially reduces the incidence of formal induction of labour."

You have the right to decline this intervention, and may want to inform yourself more about something which may seem at the time to be a better option than formal induction, but which may lead on to further intervention. See Sara Wickham's blogpost, www.sarawickham.com/research-updates/membrane-sweeping-for-induction-of-labour/

Induction of labour

"When nature does work, it cannot be improved. Technology does not enhance a natural process that is working. It can only mar or destroy it." (Stewart 1998).

Induction of labour is an increasingly common intervention. In the UK one in three (33%) women have their labours induced (NHS Digital 2019).

Induction of labour can involve sweeping the membranes, inserting a pessary into your vagina to soften your cervix, breaking your waters, and/or the use of oxytocin (syntocinon in the UK, and Pitocin in the USA and elsewhere). This is administered through a drip in your arm (when these are advised during labour it is called augmentation of labour). There are many reasons why induction of labour might be suggested. For example, if you are over 40 weeks pregnant.

According to the findings of some research, there is little evidence of benefit to support inducing women before 42 weeks (Keulen et al 2018). WHO states that:
"There is insufficient evidence to recommend induction of labour for women with uncomplicated pregnancies before 41 weeks of pregnancy" (WHO 2018a). Despite research indicating its overuse the numbers are still increasing.

The procedure, whilst helpful in certain circumstances, is not benign and *"all induced women will be exposed to potential disadvantages"* (Seijmonsbergen-Schermers et al 2019).

Whatever reason you are given, you can ask what the benefits and risks might be of an induction compared to waiting, along with the research that supports the HPs advice. You have the right to say you wish to take some time to consider the advice and that you will let your HP know your decision. You then have the opportunity to discuss this with others, and you may wish to read Sara Wickham's book *Inducing Labour – Making Informed Decisions* (2018) and Rachel Reed's book *Why Induction Matters* (2019).

For some women, an induction can be straightforward but many women do not realise that induction of labour is a major intervention which can be very painful, can sometimes take a number of days, and can involve women requiring or requesting epidural anaesthesia.

Some women ask for an induction for a variety of reasons: for example, they want their husband, or partner, to be with them and she or he will only be able to be there on a specific date; or they are finding pregnancy increasingly difficult.

The last few weeks of pregnancy allow the baby to put on weight and continue brain development to prepare for the world outside the womb, and should not be regarded lightly. One rarely mentioned disadvantage of induction is brought up by Michel Odent, who notes that the mother's antibodies are transferred to her baby by the placenta and increase rapidly after 38 weeks, *"reaching more than twice the maternal concentrations at the time of delivery."*

This raises a question about how many antibodies the baby might be deprived of if induced at 39 or 40 weeks, when he or she might have been born after 40 weeks had the induction not been carried out.

Hospital admission criteria

Most women will experience a period of *pre-labour*, where your body is softening and effacing your cervix. For some women, these sensations can feel quite strong and go on for a long time. Women can be very disheartened when they find that they are in early labour and have not reached four centimetres dilation of the cervix, the usual admission criteria to hospital (though this varies). It is during this period that many women will go to hospital, only to be sent home having been told that they are not in labour (Shallow 2019).

Many women are more comfortable labouring at home during early labour, but some women's labours can progress quickly and, occasionally, women are further on in labour than HPs realise. If you think your labour is progressing quickly, although you cannot insist on having a birthing room, you can remain on the hospital premises, or nearby, and see how your labour goes.

Amniotomy – Breaking the waters or Artificial Rupture of Membranes (ARM)

The bag of waters (amniotic sac) surrounding your baby protects it from infection during pregnancy and spreads the pressure of the contractions during labour. For many women, it will stay intact until near full dilatation when the waters may break spontaneously; in some rare cases they may not break at all, and the baby can be born within the bag of waters (the caul).

Some women might be told that the midwife *has to break the waters* because the labour is not progressing or because *it will help speed up the labour.* There is little evidence to support this, and introducing an instrument into your vagina can increase the risk of infection, but some women may get relief, and find that their labour does progress. Others might experience decreased confidence in their bodies, and increased pain as their baby's head presses directly on their cervix, necessitating an epidural or other pain relieving drugs. In very rare cases, the umbilical cord can be swept down the birth canal ahead of the baby (a cord prolapse). This usually necessitates immediate surgery, a caesarean. If this were to happen at home an immediate hospital transfer would be required.

As with every other intervention, you have the right to decline having your waters broken.

Electronic Fetal Heart monitoring (EFM)

Electronic fetal heart monitoring, also called a cardiotocograph or CTG, is commonly used in the UK and many other countries when women arrive in hospital in labour, and during labour. It uses ultrasound to monitor the baby's heartbeat and involves strapping the monitoring device (transducer) to the woman's abdomen. As a result, the woman is usually expected to lie on a bed – though it can be used with women standing, kneeling or sitting and some practitioners encourage this. There are monitors that use wireless monitoring (telemetry), that enable you to walk around or adopt other positions. These are not universally available or used, though you can ask your HPs about their availability. It is unclear whether it improves outcomes for mothers and babies with potential or actual complications (Small et al 2019).

A critical paper by Sartwelle and Johnson (2015) points out that EFM is *"based on 19th-century childbirth myths, a virtually non-existent scientific foundation, and has a false positive rate exceeding 99%."* (See also Sara Wickham, *The case against electronic fetal monitoring*, 2020).

Electronic Fetal Heart Monitoring (EFM) during labour

Despite Sartwelle and Johnson's criticisms, many hospitals advise women to have continuous electronic fetal monitoring for at least twenty minutes when they get to hospital in labour. The Cochrane summary of admission CTG vs intermittent monitoring concludes that, *"Although many hospitals carry out CTGs on women when they are admitted to hospital in labour, we found no evidence that this benefits women with low-risk pregnancies. We found that admission CTGs may increase numbers of women having a caesarean section by about 20%."* (Devane et al 2017).

You have the right to decline any offer to have an admission CTG trace and you can ask for the baby's heartbeat to be listened to intermittently – with a Pinard stethoscope or a hand-held Doppler monitor.

A Cochrane review compared continuous EFM with intermittent auscultation, listening to the baby's heart beat every 15 minutes or so during labour, and found that when EFM was used there was a reduction in the neonatal seizure rate but no significant differences in cerebral palsy or infant mortality. EFM was, however, associated with an increase in caesarean surgery and instrumental vaginal births (Alfirevic et al 2017).

"In randomised clinical trials comparing electronic monitoring with intermittent auscultation, electronic monitoring increased the risk of caesarean by 63%. This suggests that, if electronic monitoring had not been used in those 620,000 women, 240,000 fewer of them would have had caesarean deliveries." (Nelson et al 2016).

When EFM was used during preterm labour, it was associated with a higher incidence of cerebral palsy (Small et al 2020).

It is concerning that repeated reviews of EFM invariably comment on the poor quality of the research evidence reviewed, and call for yet more research rather than reducing its use.

If HPs suggest that you should be continuously monitored you can ask why, and for how long. You have the right to decline or you could ask for your labour to be monitored intermittently, which the midwife can do with a Pinard stethoscope, or a hand held monitor which uses Doppler ultrasound.

Vaginal Examinations (VEs)

The use of routine vaginal examinations varies across the UK and elsewhere. In some areas VEs are advised on admission to hospital in labour, every two to four hours during labour, and before a woman gets into a birth pool. In some areas, HPs are being encouraged to carry out few, or no, vaginal examinations unless they are necessary and the HP cannot gain necessary information any other way. In these circumstances, a vaginal examination might help a practitioner make useful suggestions about positions you might adopt and/or help you and your HP make decisions about your labour. There is little good evidence to support the routine use of VEs. Women can find them uncomfortable or distressing and they increase the risk of infection: *"It is surprising that there is such a widespread use of this intervention without good evidence of its effectiveness, particularly considering the sensitivity of the procedure for the women receiving it, and the potential for adverse consequences in some settings."* (Downe et al 2013). They can be particularly painful and distressing if women have had their labours induced with prostaglandin pessaries and/or have suffered sexual abuse.

A VE only provides a snapshot in time as your cervix can dilate or shrink, and it may be that the stress of the examination itself causes your cervix to close. VEs can also reduce a woman's confidence in giving birth, particularly if, for example, after an examination she is told that she is *only* x centimetres dilated or has *a long way to go yet*.

If you have an induced or accelerated labour, you will usually be offered VEs at regular intervals during labour. The decision whether to accept or decline is yours, but they may be necessary if, for example, you want an epidural.

There are alternative methods of determining the progress of the labour, which skilled midwives know about and use. One example that can be used along with other signs of progress is:
"The presence of a purple line during labour, seen to rise from the anal margin and extend between the buttocks as labour progresses has been reported." (Shepherd et al 2010).

A study in Iran (Kordi et al 2014) concluded that, as the appearance of the purple line is a very accurate predictor of the progression of labour, *"we can use it as a non-invasive complementary method for clinical assessment of labor progress at clinics."* (See also Sara Wickham's blog *Evidence for the purple line* 2014). However, this is rarely used as most NHS trusts do not currently see it as valid.

Whatever your circumstances, you can ask why a VE is being advised, the evidence to justify this, and what alternatives there are. You can also ask for the VE to be conducted with you in a different position, perhaps on your hands and knees, if lying on your back is too painful. Or you can decline some or all VEs.

Birth positions

Few women instinctively want to lie down during labour and birth. Many women will give birth on their hands and knees or other upright positions if they are encouraged to follow their instincts (Edwards 2019). These positions allow your pelvis to open and use gravity to help your baby be born more easily. You can give birth in any position you choose and you do not have to lie on your back or have your feet in stirrups, unless you agree that there is a good reason for this to be suggested. Professor Roberto Caldeyro Barcia, past President of the International Federation of Obstetricians and Gynaecologists, once commented that: *"There is only one position worse than laying on your back for the birth, it is hanging by your heels from a chandelier."* (Personal communication 1985).

Research has clearly demonstrated that women have easier labours, fewer epidurals and less risk of having caesarean surgery if they are able to move around and adopt positions in which they feel comfortable (Lawrence et al 2013).

A Cochrane review of upright positions for birth found that when women give birth on their backs, there is a greater liklihood of the use of forceps, or an episiotomy (Gupta et al 2017).

A Care Quality Commission report, however, shockingly revealed that over one in five women (22%) having a *normal* birth did so in obstetric stirrups (Care Quality Commission 2018).

You can give birth in any position you want, and many practitioners encourage this and provide mats on the floor, birth balls, pillows, bars on the wall and other equipment to facilitate upright positions.

Eating and drinking

"Women should be free to eat and drink in labour, or not, as they wish." (Singata et al 2013)

Labour is hard work and you need to eat and drink as you want during that time. If you are prevented from doing so during your labour, your body will try and find energy from another source. If it does this for too long, you can become ketotic. This is when your body cannot get enough glucose from the blood and begins to burn fat. This condition is often resolved by putting up a glucose drip, instead of encouraging you to eat and drink in the first place.

In the past, anaesthetists would insist that women should not eat during labour because of the risks of inhaling vomit if they were to be anaesthetised.

The Cochrane Review of fluid and food intake during labour concludes that: *"there is no justification for the restriction of fluids and food in labour for women at low risk of complications."* (Singata et al 2013).

All hospitals can provide water for women in labour and in some areas women are encouraged to eat and drink as they want. A few birth centres even provide food, but some hospitals may still seek to restrict food intake in labour. You have the right to eat and drink as you feel inclined, and it is always a good idea to have some food of your choice with you, at home or in hospital, especially if you are in hospital for an extended period. At home, you can eat and drink as you wish. Many women eat less, or nothing, as labour progresses, but continue to drink herbal teas with honey, nutritious drinks or iced water, and some women feel sick or vomit as labour progresses.

Time limits

The findings of research increasingly support women being able to labour and birth in their own time and way. Many practitioners are trying to change hospital policies and guidelines to reflect this evidence.

The majority of UK hospitals, in common with those in many other countries, however, still have variations of active management of labour (AML) in place. This is where labour is required to fit within specific time limits, and if it does not, various interventions are advised to ensure that it does. These artificial time limits often create a sense of urgency which interferes with the birth process, and which can increase interventions (Murphy-Lawless 1998 and Edwards 2019).

Midwifery models, knowledge and practices, are less reliant on time and are based more on gauging how each individual woman and baby are doing, and whether or not progress is being made. Experienced midwives recognise that some labours may only last two hours, others may last over 24 hours, but supporting women having long, but normal, labours can be difficult if guidelines suggest intervening.

If there are time limits in place where you are giving birth and you are told that you are *not progressing*, you do not have to accept interventions. You can ask whether or not there is a problem with you or your baby, then consider how you feel. If you and your baby are well, and you feel that you are coping, you can decide that no action be taken at the moment and suggest considering a review in a couple of hours.

Pain relief

Many women worry about whether or not they are going to be able to cope with the pain of labour. Those who feel private, safe, and supported, release pain relieving hormones, known as endorphins, and may find using their breath, vocalising, being mobile, using a birth pool, bath or shower, massage, aromatherapy, hypnobirthing and/or a TENS machine, helpful in enabling them to feel calm and to release more endorphins. Some women report that they found labour orgasmic. (Buckley 2015).

If you need additional pain relief, especially if your labour has been induced or accelerated, or if you are lying on your back being continuously monitored, which can increase the pain of labour, you can use gas and air, at home or in hospital, a variety of analgesics, or an epidural, which is only available in obstetric units. Interventions disrupt the normal flow of hormones that ease labour, and remove women's coping strategies, such as being mobile.

Some women are so anxious that they want to book an epidural in early labour in the hope that they will avoid any pain. You can request or decline any form of pain relief during labour, but if you wish to avoid pharmaceutical pain relief you may want to put this in your birth plan, have someone with you who is aware of this, and tell your HP that you will request it if you need it, but would rather not be offered it.

Epidural anaesthesia

If you need, or decide to have, caesarean surgery you will find that the majority are undertaken with a spinal or epidural anaesthetic. The risks are lower than the risks of a general anaesthetic, and you can be conscious, and your baby will be exposed to lower amounts of medication

If you need pharmacological pain relief during labour, an epidural is a very effective form of pain relief, which works most of the time. A study by Kingsley (2017) found an epidural failure or partial failure rate of approximately 9-12%.

Epidurals can, however, influence the course of labour and birth. They can, for example, increase the length of labour (Cheng 2014) and the likelihood of more forceps or ventouse deliveries (Anim-Somuah et al 2018). They are also only available in an obstetric unit.

Henci Goer's article analysing the question about whether or not epidurals increase the risk of caesarean section concluded that, *"At the very least we cannot assure women with confidence that epidurals don't increase the likelihood of caesarean."* (Goer 2015).

A more recent, systematic review of randomised controlled trials of epidural use in labour revealed that much of the epidural research is of low quality (Anim-Somuah et al 2018).

Women who have had an epidural in place for more than six hours can have an increase in temperature, which may indicate a fever (see Buckley 2005). If that occurs, HPs are likely to worry about the possibility of you having an infection, which you may or may not have, and then consider giving antibiotics to both you and your baby.

Occasionally women suffer what is called a *dural tap*. This happens when, instead of the epidural needle going into the epidural space, it accidentally punctures the dural sac, which contains spinal fluid. The fluid then leaks out causing a severe headache, which the Royal College of Anaesthetists estimates occurs between 1 in 100 and 1 in 500 cases. Usually, you will then be expected to lie flat for some time, which makes caring for a newborn baby difficult, and can delay your discharge from hospital often by two to three days.

As with any pain relief, it is your right to accept or decline the offer of an epidural, but accepting an epidural may mean that other interventions, for example vaginal examination, become more necessary, to ensure that the baby is not just about to be born.

Meconium staining

Some babies pass meconium before or during labour, especially if they are over 40 weeks gestation. This is the baby's first bowel movement. The implications of meconium staining can depend upon the type of meconium, and the condition and gestation of the baby. Rarely, passing meconium in labour can have serious adverse effects on the baby. In most cases it will not (Davies 2011, Edwards 2019, Powell 2013, Reed 2015).

In Silke Powell's article on meconium she points out that, *"most infants with a poor outcome do not pass meconium in labour"* and *"most babies exposed to meconium liquor are born in good condition."* She later comments: *"... there is increasing evidence to support the theory that meconium is passed in utero as a result of the physiological maturation of the fetal gastrointestinal tract. In other words, it's a normal process."* (Powell 2013).

When this happens, however, you will usually be strongly advised to have continuous electronic fetal heart monitoring. This is your decision. If you are at home you will be advised strongly to transfer to hospital for continuous electronic fetal heart monitoring and so that the baby has access to other equipment if needed. A transfer may not be needed, and it is your decision whether or not to move, although it may be difficult to make that decision, especially if you can't get a second opinion.

If you have been advised, or told, to give birth in a consultant unit, because of meconium staining during your last labour, you have the right to accept or decline that advice.

When a baby needs resuscitation

Some babies (especially those born early, those of low birth weight, or with health problems) do not breathe easily after birth and may need resuscitating. Sometimes the baby is taken to another room where there is more specialised resuscitation equipment, and the father or birth partner can accompany the baby. Some hospitals are adopting resuscitation trolleys that can be used alongside you, so that treatment can be done without cutting the umbilical cord early and to avoid separating you from your baby. You can ask about what usually happens in your local hospital and, if resuscitation trolleys are not available, you could suggest this to the senior obstetrician, senior midwife, the local MVP or MSLC.

Birthing your placenta

Until recently it was routine practice to inject a drug into your thigh, as your baby's shoulder emerged. This was to speed up the birth of the placenta and prevent you losing too much blood, to clamp and cut the cord immediately after your baby's birth, and to pull out the placenta. If, however, you have had a labour and birth without drugs, or other interventions, routinely managing the birth of the placenta may not be needed. If, however, your labour has been induced or augmented there is an increased risk of haemorrhage, and this is a good reason for managing the birth of the placenta with drugs (Edwards and Wickham 2018). You can decide beforehand how you want to birth your placenta, but may want to change your mind depending on how birth unfolds.

A normal or physiological birth of the placenta can take 40 minutes or more after the birth of your baby (Dixon et al 2009), although in some, now very unusual, circumstances it could take a few hours.

"We waited two hours until the cord stopped pulsing." (Linton 2017).

I recall being told of a woman who gave birth on a yacht crossing the Pacific; the placenta finally arrived over 24 hours later.

Having your baby nuzzle, lick at your breast, or breastfeed, can increase the flow of oxytocin which causes uterine contractions which help release your placenta. Trying to have a pee sometimes helps to deliver the placenta, as a full bladder can inhibit the placenta's descent. HPs may have other helpful suggestions for birthing your placenta, if you are not bleeding too much, and your placenta has separated from the uterine wall but is just taking time.

Clamping and cutting the baby's umbilical cord

Until recently, it has been accepted practice in many countries for the cord to be clamped routinely within a minute or so of your baby's birth, despite there being no evidence to support this intervention. The umbilical cord provides your baby with essential nutrients, blood, oxygen, antibodies and stem cells, and continues to do so after your baby has been born, providing the cord is not clamped until it stops pulsating – to clamp early deprives your baby of these essential benefits (Burleigh 2012, Edwards and Wickham 2018).

The Resuscitation Council guidelines recommend *"a delay in cord clamping of at least one minute"* but this seems to be an arbitrary time as the guidelines don't cite any research evidence to justify this early intervention. (Wyllie 2015).

There is no need to clamp and cut the cord unless you want to or, for example, if the cord is too short to enable you to hold and/or feed your baby easily.

Midwives have observed that leaving the cord until it stops pulsating, preferably until it is thin and white, can take anything from a few minutes to half an hour.

If you give birth at home, and if your baby arrives before the midwives, the cord should be left unclamped and intact. Keep your baby warm by holding him or her skin to skin, with a blanket or towel over both you and baby, as newborn babies can otherwise get cold very quickly.

Most areas have introduced delayed cord clamping but a survey of parents' views on this intervention showed that while 75% requested a delay, either in their birth plan or during labour, 20% reported that the cord was clamped immediately (Positive Birth Movement 2018).

You have a right to inform the midwife or doctor that the cord should not be clamped and cut until you decide otherwise.

Cord blood collection

Some hospitals have given commercial and charitable companies access to labour wards in order to seek parents' permission to collect volumes of umbilical cord blood immediately after their baby's birth.

Charitable companies rely on the altruism of parents by advertising that if they donate the umbilical cord blood, which they describe as a waste product, they will be helping save lives. These companies have targets of 150mls per baby to reach. There is no evidence to say that this is safe for the baby. Parents need to be fully informed of the research that recommends a delay of 3-5 minutes is optimal, as earlier clamping can impact on neurological development.

Commercial companies inform parents that they can store their baby's stem cells in case they become ill with a range of disorders at a later date. This method usually includes clamping at one minute. Some companies will delay for longer, but this will affect the amount of cord blood obtained. Technological advances have meant that one company states that a smaller amount of blood after optimal cord clamping would be sufficient.

The blood in the umbilical cord and placenta is a rich source of stem cells and, following birth, these stem cells migrate to different parts of your baby's system. These cells are your baby's building blocks for life. Early clamping deprives your baby of over a million stem cells and we do not know the long-term effects of this deprivation.

Many hospitals clamp and cut the cord at one minute, as NICE guidance states that 1-5 minutes is sufficient. The latest research states that at least 3 or 5, and even 10 minutes, is the minimum time the cord should be clamped.

Early clamping can deprive your baby of around 30% of their total blood. Studies show that for term babies having a normal vaginal birth, the babies will lose on average 100mls, but other estimates range between 60 to 240mls (Dawes 1968).

Optimal cord clamping affords the baby a natural physiological transition. This can take a varying amount of time, and the HP should be looking to support a physiological transition by looking at baby rather than watching the clock. Any potential donation or storage of cord blood should be considered after the baby has safely transited to extra uterine life and not before. HPs should also ensure parents are giving fully informed consent, especially in the light of the strong evidence to support a longer delay than 1 minute, and the potential detrimental effect on neurological development.

"Paediatric guidelines state that 'blood draws in infants and children should not exceed 5% of the total blood volume in any 24-hour period'. A 3.6kg new-born has a blood volume of around 280mls – so the maximum blood draw would be 14mls" ... *"The minimum amount of blood*

acceptable for collection is 45mls, and the maximum possible is 215mls." (Reed, 2020 see also Burleigh, 2020).

It is possible to donate your baby's blood, after the cord has stopped pulsating, as the company can collect the umbilical cord and the placenta and drain the blood from them. You may wish to donate your baby's blood in this way, but you also have a right to decline.

Lotus birth

A Lotus birth is where the umbilical cord and placenta are left alone until the cord detaches itself from the baby – usually after about three days. You have the right to insist that the cord is not cut and that you will be keeping the cord and placenta attached to the baby until it falls off naturally (see Resources, website –Ted Talk).

Who owns your placenta?

Your placenta, or afterbirth, is your property.

If you give birth in hospital, you can leave the placenta's disposal to the hospital, as many women do. You also have the right to take the placenta home with you if you wish to. If you give birth at home, the midwife will usually take the placenta away for disposal, but you can keep it. Some women bury it in the garden under a rose bush or tree. Occasionally women eat some of the placenta, cooked, raw or encapsulated (dried and made into small pills). They believe that it benefits them physically and emotionally, postnatally, due to its high levels of hormones. Most animals eat their placenta after birth, probably so as not to draw attention to their young. There is no research to support or refute the benefits or otherwise of eating or encapsulating the placenta for new mothers.

Premature, low birth weight or ill babies

If your baby is born prematurely, is of low birth weight and/or unwell, this can be a shock and extremely distressing, especially if this is unexpected. It can feel as though decisions are being made for you and that you have less contact with your baby than you want. There are positive things you can do for your baby in these circumstances. Many benefits have been found for skin-to-skin contact: for example, the growth of low birth-weight babies is improved (Suman 2008). It also results in more women breastfeeding up to four months after the birth (Moore et al 2016).

Additionally, a mother who sang to her premature baby during kangaroo care reduced maternal anxiety and stabilised the baby (Arnon et al 2014).

Research shows that babies regulate their temperature better when they are placed next to their mother's skin or between her breasts rather than in an incubator; it also has the added advantage of providing easily accessible breast milk (see *Kangaroo Babies: A different way of mothering* by Charpak and Powell (2016), and *The Positive Breastfeeding Book* by Amy Brown 2019).

If regulation of your baby's temperature is the only reason for advising that s/he be taken to the special care baby unit, you can insist that the baby stays skin to skin, and if HPs do not agree, ask for the consultant paediatrician to attend to discuss this with you.

When a baby needs neonatal care

If your baby needs neonatal care, the father or birth partner has a right to accompany him/her if you are unable to do so, so that you can then be informed of what has happened. For practical reasons, parents could be excluded in an emergency, but the doctors and nurses still have a duty to consult with parents and keep you fully informed of your baby's treatment. You can usually still touch, talk and sing to your baby when they are receiving neonatal care.

This chapter has covered the more common issues that you might want to think and make decisions about. Whatever the suggested course of action, you have the right to ask for detailed information about the advantages and disadvantages of following it, and you have the right to accept or decline any suggested course of action or treatment.

Chapter 8
After the Birth

This chapter addresses some of the issues that may arise once you have had your baby, and what your options are. Some are rare and specific, some routine, but whatever issues you face as a parent, you have the right to information, advice and support, and the right to accept treatment for your baby; and in all but the most urgent of situations, the right to decline treatment for your baby.

Postnatal care is crucial for the wellbeing and health of both mother and baby, but this is not routinely provided in all countries (such as the USA), and the provision varies between countries and regions. Unfortunately, postnatal care is not seen as a priority, despite the numbers of mothers and babies who have developed serious problems, which could have been detected and treated earlier had the midwives been enabled to provide the standard of care that they are trained for and want to provide (the restrictions imposed by Covid-19 have further restricted the provision of postnatal care in many areas).

At one time, midwives in the UK were required, and able, to visit every day for ten days after the birth before handing over to a health visitor. If a midwife was concerned about a mother and baby, or felt they needed more support, she could extend this to 28 days. In many areas there is a desperate shortage of both hospital and community midwives and they no longer have the resources to do this. In some areas, midwives will check how you and your baby are doing mainly by telephone. This puts both women and babies at risk, particularly when nearly one in three women will have had caesarean surgery. Many women suffer from postnatal depression or trauma and many will need breastfeeding support. The findings of numerous studies have revealed women's dissatisfaction with the quality of postnatal services, both in hospital and in the community. The CQC's survey of women's experiences postnatally noted that *"just over a fifth (21%) of women reported that they would have liked to have seen a midwife more often."* (Care Quality

Commission 2018). A similar survey in Scotland found that women indicated *"how vitally important it is for them to have the opportunity to develop relationships with staff through continuity of care."* (Cheyne 2015). Similar views were expressed by women in Northern Ireland and Wales.

If, however, after your baby is born, you wish to see a midwife, you can ask her to visit each day, until you are feeling better or more confident, or you can phone the Community Midwives' office to request support. You can also phone the postnatal ward of your local hospital for support and information. Each area will have its own system so check what is available in your hospital.

Checking your baby

"Newborns without complications should be kept in skin-to-skin contact (SSC) with their mothers during the first hour after birth to prevent hypothermia and promote breastfeeding" (WHO 2018b).

Many practitioners understand the benefits of, and promote, skin-to-skin contact between a mother and her newborn immediately after birth. Many mothers make it clear in their birth plans that they want their baby placed on their tummies, or pick the baby up themselves, so that they can spend some time holding and saying hello to the baby and having skin-to-skin contact.

If your baby is born early, and/or is small, or you have had a caesarean, skin-to-skin contact is particularly beneficial as it improves growth and development (Suman 2008), improved blood flow to the heart and brain (Sehgal et al 2020), and more women were breastfeeding up to four months after the birth (Moore et al 2016).

After you have welcomed your baby, the midwife will want to check and weigh him/her. If your baby is healthy, there is no urgency to do this and she should seek your permission to do so. A midwife or doctor does not have the right to remove a baby without a parent's consent.

Between six and 72 hours, a baby should receive a more detailed neonatal examination by a suitably trained midwife, nurse, GP, or paediatrician, so that any problems may be detected and treated. A further check should also be offered between six and eight weeks following the birth, by the woman's GP.

Many midwives are trained to do the neonatal examination shortly after the birth. For information about the neonatal examination after a home birth see Chapter 4, Home Births. For more information about what the postnatal check involves. (see Resources, Websites – Postnatal check)

Feeding your baby

During your pregnancy you may make a decision about how you want to feed your baby. Whether you decide to breastfeed, formula feed or combination feed, the decision is yours. Some mothers leave the decision until after they have given birth. However you decide to feed your baby, you should be given accurate information and support for your chosen method.

During the early phases of the pandemic, some hospitals decided to isolate the baby if the mother tested positive for Covid-19, despite a WHO recommendation that mothers with suspected or confirmed Covid-19 *"should be enabled to remain together while rooming-in throughout the day and night and to practice skin-to-skin contact, including kangaroo mother care especially immediately after birth and during establishment of breastfeeding."* (WHO 2020).

Isolating a baby can result in stress for the mother and baby and have adverse long-term consequences for bonding, breastfeeding, and the baby's immune system (Stuebe 2020). You have the right to refuse to be separated from your baby and ask the HPs to produce the evidence they have for their proposed intervention.

Women are currently often told very firmly by HPs that they must not share a bed, or co-sleep, with their baby as it is a dangerous practice. This is a very clear example of the over-extension of a rule that is appropriate for a minority of women but not necessarily for those who breastfeed, know the rules of safer sleeping, and don't smoke, drink excessively or take other drugs. Many women continue to co-sleep, following the example of women around the world, but are afraid to confess this to HPs.

NICE has recently issued new guidance highlighting the fact that professionals should discuss safer co-sleeping and any risks with parents-to-be during pregnancy and the postnatal period. Amy Brown, in her book, *Breastfeeding Uncovered*, gives a very clear account of the benefits and risks of the different places that babies can sleep as well as the beneficial effect of co-sleeping on breastfeeding rates.

Breastfeeding

Breastfeeding has long-term benefits: it can reduce your baby's risk of infections and cardiovascular disease in adulthood; it can also lower your risk of breast and ovarian cancer, cardiovascular disease, and osteoporosis, even if you only breastfeed for a short time.

Avoiding formula milk for at least the first three days of your baby's life decreases the incidence of sensitisation to cows' milk and clinical food allergies (Urashima et al 2019). However, many women find breastfeeding difficult, and some feel guilty that they are not able to provide breastmilk for their baby (Brown 2018).

Many women do not realise that if they have had obstetric interventions, and/or drugs, these can have a significant effect on the baby. The result is often a sleepy or fractious baby, who is not very interested in feeding; combine that with lack of support, anxiety, and pressure to give the baby formula, it is not surprising that many women stop breastfeeding before they want to.

The Care Quality Commission reported that:
"almost 34% of women reported not being encouraged to breastfeed their babies within the first hour after birth".

It also reported: *"evidence of poor breastfeeding support for multiparous mothers* [those who have previously given birth] *and that out of 80% of women who wanted to breastfeed, only 57% reported that they received enough information."* (Care Quality Commission Survey 2018).

If your baby is not yet ready or is unable to breastfeed directly, you should be able to obtain a hospital grade pump from the maternity unit to express your milk, which can be given to your baby in a cup; or it can be frozen and stored until it can be used. This also helps to maintain your milk supply.

If you are unable, for whatever reason, to provide enough of your own milk, you can ask the hospital to source screened and processed donor breast milk from an NHS milk bank. More information about donor breast milk is available from the UK Association for Milk Banking and for helpline information (see Resources, Organisations).

Sometimes women whose babies have spent time in special, or intensive care, discover that the HPs have given the baby a bottle of formula food or water without asking for their consent. No health practitioner has the right to give your baby any food or liquid without your consent and UNICEF warns that *"Unnecessary supplementation with infant formula will interfere with [...] physiology, resulting in less frequent feeds. Introducing infant formula changes the gut flora of the baby, making them more susceptible to infections and/or allergies and can also undermine a mother's confidence in her ability to breastfeed."* (UNICEF 2020). This is an assault, and you have every right to make a complaint about the HP's failure to consult you before feeding your baby.

If you are not receiving the breastfeeding support you need, you do not have to struggle on alone. You can see if a local volunteer breastfeeding counsellor can help, or your hospital's infant feeding co-ordinator, if they have one, or you might need to find a local Lactation Consultant. Most NHS hospitals, and NHS UK, provide information online about what breastfeeding support there is, so you can see what there is available in your area. Alternatively, see the resources section for other sources of information and support.

Vitamin K

The recommendation in the UK is for all babies to receive a dose of Vitamin K, to prevent a rare condition called haemorrhagic disease of the newborn (excessive bleeding). Usually it is given shortly after birth by injection, but it can be given by mouth, if this is what you decide. The rationale for this recommendation is based on looking at the levels of vitamin K that babies are born with and the measured levels in breast milk alongside the fact that 1 in 11,000 babies in high income countries who do not receive Vitamin K can be affected by late onset Vitamin K deficiency bleeding.

It can be argued that routine Vitamin K for babies at risk is of value, but questions have been raised about its routine use and any potential risks. The decision whether or not to give Vitamin K can be complex. For a comprehensive discussion of the issues read Sara Wickham's book *Vitamin K and the Newborn* (2017).

Most parents agree to Vitamin K for their babies, but parents have the right to refuse administration of Vitamin K. Some HPs are insistent that all babies should be given Vitamin K, and sometimes refer parents to a paediatrician, if they are unable to *persuade* the parents to agree to it. Occasionally, HPs have threatened to report the parents to social services.

A referral to social services should only be made if there is a risk of significant harm to the baby. Refusing the administration of Vitamin K is not grounds for a referral, and anyone who makes such threats should be reported to the hospital's Chief Executive and also to the Nursing and Midwifery Council or the General Medical Council.

If you have been threatened in this way, you can seek help from your local or national support groups (see Resources, Organisations).

The NHS Newborn Blood Spot (NBS) Screening formerly known as the Guthrie Test

Four or five days after your baby is born you will be offered a blood test for your baby. This involves pricking the baby's heel to obtain a blood spot for testing. This is used to identify those babies who have phenylketonuria (PKU), a rare inherited enzyme deficiency that occurs in the UK in about 1 in 10,000 babies, but can vary in different populations. The blood is also tested for a range of other conditions, such as: congenital hypothyroidism, cystic fibrosis, sickle cell disease and MCAD (Medium Chain acyl-CoA Dehydrogenase Deficiency).

Research has shown that babies tolerate blood tests and injections far better if they are held in their mother's arms and breastfed while this is undertaken (Harrison et al 2020). One mother commented:

"Other than a bit of clamping down when the needle went in, the babe carried on feeding undisturbed and there was no crying at all."

Suckling from a bottle can produce a similarly soothing effect during the blood spot test.

Your consent is required before this test is carried out, and you have the right to accept or decline.

When there is a disagreement

As soon as your baby is born, you assume parental rights.

"If the parents of a child are married when the child is born, or if they've jointly adopted a child, both have parental responsibility." (Gov.uk 2020).

All health professionals want to act in the best interests of the mother and her baby, and generally parents and HPs work together well, but sometimes parents feel that the treatment that is proposed is not appropriate, and express their concern, oppose its continuation or want alternative treatments.

You have every right to require the HP to justify the reasons for the proposed treatment. If the disagreement is not resolved by discussion, you have a right to ask for a more senior member of staff to attend, or to ask for a second opinion from elsewhere.

If the HP considers that without appropriate treatment the baby is at risk, and the parents disagree with this advice, the staff have the right to apply for a Court Order to keep the baby in the special care baby unit and carry out the treatment they are recommending.

If you do not agree with the treatment the health practitioners intend implementing, you can insist that your disagreement is recorded in the baby's case notes.

Occasionally, HPs have threatened parents with reporting them to social services, or calling the police. Should this occur the parents can contact their local or national support groups for advice and assistance (see Resources, Organisations); and it would be wise to make notes of any conversations or, even better, record them.

If the baby needs to be transferred to a different hospital

If your baby needs treatment that cannot be provided at the hospital where you gave birth, your baby will be transferred to another hospital with appropriate facilities. It is customary for the mother to accompany the baby, although it may not always be possible for you to travel in the ambulance, because of the large amount of equipment that may have to be carried as well, or you may not be well enough to travel. If transfer is needed shortly after the birth, the hospital will make arrangements for the parents to follow. Parents should not be expected to make their own way to the new hospital within hours or days of the birth.

If twins, or more, have been born, it is possible that the babies could be transferred to different hospitals, which can be particularly stressful for parents and make contact more difficult.

When to leave hospital

After having a baby, women were once expected to stay in hospital for up to 14 days after the birth. Some women could not leave soon enough, but others welcomed the break from the demands of home and/or appreciated the help they received with breastfeeding and care of their baby. Nowadays, in the UK, *"women are most likely to stay in hospital for one to two days (36%), followed by women who stay more than 12 hours but less than 24 hours (21%), and those staying only up to 12 hours (17%). Most women think that the length of their stay was about right (72%)."* (Care Quality Commission 2018).

You have the right to leave hospital with your baby once you feel ready, unless a HP has legitimate concerns about your baby's health, but if you feel you need to stay longer you can discuss this with a HP.

Leaving hospital against medical advice

Most women are encouraged and supported to leave hospital after birth as soon as they feel ready. You have the right to leave hospital with your baby once you feel ready, although if a HP has concerns about the baby's health you may be told that the baby must stay. Strictly, a court order would be needed to compel either a mother or her baby to stay or be kept in hospital but in practice it is very difficult, as well as unusual, for a woman to insist on taking her baby home if there are serious and legitimate concerns about the baby.

Many hospitals ask the mother to sign a disclaimer if she wants to leave against the advice of HPs, usually titled *Discharge against medical advice*. There is no obligation to sign a discharge form, but if you decide to do so you have the right to write your reasons for leaving, so that the hospital management will be aware of your reasons for taking an early discharge. You can ask for a photocopy for any future reference, or take a photograph of the form yourself.

If HPs insist that you and your baby must stay for a longer period, and you disagree, you can ask them to put their reasons for this advice in writing first. If they are not willing to do so, you might conclude that they do not have legitimate grounds for persuading you to stay.

A woman's right to stay in hospital

Current lack of resources, and high numbers of women giving birth in many of our busy hospitals, can put pressure on HPs to discharge women from hospital as soon as possible after birth. Some women may feel that they need additional support and do not want to leave hospital early and midwives will do their best to accommodate you if you need more support.

If you have had a difficult birth, or caesarean surgery, you may not feel well enough to return home. You may also be without support at home. You can insist on staying until you feel fit enough to cope with your newborn baby at home, and if you still feel under pressure to go home, you should ask to see the Director/Head of Midwifery to discuss this.

Notifying and registering your baby's birth

Birth notification

At a home or hospital birth, in the UK, the attending midwife has a legal responsibility to notify the local hospital's or the Health Board's Child Health Department of the birth so that your baby will have an NHS number.

If you give birth without a midwife or doctor present, and the midwives do not visit you within 6 hours, then normally it is the father's responsibility to inform the Child Health Department. The notification can also be made in writing within 36 hours of the baby's birth (Notification of Births Act 1907).

Birth registration

Irrespective of place of birth, parents in England and Wales have a legal responsibility to register the birth of their baby within 42 days of the birth (21 days in Scotland and Northern Ireland). Parents should visit the Registrar of Births, Marriages and Deaths, in the local council area in which the baby was born, to do so. One Registrar refused to register a baby's birth because the parents had not yet obtained the baby's NHS number from the Child Health Department. The requirements for birth registration are set out in the *Births and Deaths Registration Act 1953 Section 1*. This does not specify that an NHS number is necessary. A registrar who demands an NHS number before registering a birth is acting unlawfully and in breach of her or his statutory duty.

If the baby's parents are not married and the father wishes to have parental responsibility, he must be included on the birth certificate, so both parents will need to go to the Registrar of Births to do so.

This also applies if unmarried parents want the baby to have the father's surname, if not, the mother can choose to register the birth without the child's father if they're not married or in a civil partnership.

Am I Allowed: 4th Edition

Chapter 9
Making a Complaint About Your Care

The decision about whether or not, and how, to make a complaint is not an easy one for most women. Many women decide, as an alternative to making a formal complaint, to simply give feedback to the Maternity Services, hoping to improve the service for other women. This can be both satisfactory for the woman and welcomed by the service. This chapter makes suggestions about how to go about making a complaint if you decide to do this, but it is also important to have supportive others to help you through what can be a lengthy and challenging process.

Most women are satisfied with the care they receive during childbearing but, if you are dissatisfied with the care you or your baby have received, you have the right to complain. Ideally, you should do so within a year of the incident.

Before embarking on a complaint you can ask yourself the question: *"What will be the best action for me to take?"*

Many women feel that they need to get on with their lives and put the experience behind them; or they feel that if they do make a complaint little will change. Other women feel that they need to speak out about what happened in order to prevent other women suffering the same. It can be challenging dealing with the complaints procedures but lay organisations, such as AIMS, BirthRights and the Patients Association offer information, help and support (see Resources, Organisations).

Obtaining a copy of your case notes

If you decide to complain, it is important to apply in writing for a copy of your case notes.

The Data Protection Act (2018) defines General Data Protection Regulation (GDPR) giving you the right to obtain a copy of your own

False or incorrect information

If you find that information written or recorded digitally in your case notes is false or incorrect, you have the right to ask for it to be amended or removed. The Information Commissioner's Office (2020) states: *"The GDPR includes a right for individuals to have inaccurate personal data rectified, or completed if it is incomplete."*

If a hospital's Health Records Manager refuses to comply, you can insist that your letter requesting amendment or removal of information is retained in your case notes together with the response from the author of the disputed entry.

You may also have grounds to complain to the Information Commissioner, but you need to do so within three months of the last meaningful contact with the staff dealing with your complaint.

You may also wish to make a complaint to a HP's professional regulatory body. For complaints about:
- midwives, nurses, and health visitors – contact the Nursing and Midwifery Council;
- doctors – contact the General Medical Council;
- social workers – contact Social Work England, the Scottish Social Services Council, the Northern Ireland Social Care Council or Social Care Wales, depending upon where you live.

Note: The NMC Code of Practice requires HPs to *"complete records accurately and without any falsification, taking immediate and appropriate action if you become aware that someone has not kept to these requirements."* (NMC 2018).

Your right to obtain statistical information

All hospitals produce statistics, although the quality varies between hospitals. If you are making a complaint, it may be worth obtaining the statistics for the issue about which you are complaining. For example, if you felt your caesarean was unnecessary, it would be worthwhile obtaining the statistics for caesarean rates and outcomes and, if the hospital keeps them, statistics specific to a named obstetrician as some obstetricians do more caesareans than others – though it's worth bearing in mind that some obstetricians might be caring for particular groups of women who might be more likely to need or want caesarean surgery.

Your future options

Once you have a copy of your case notes you have a number of options should you still be unhappy about your care. You may feel that you would prefer to have a meeting and discuss your experiences. In which case you can:
- inform your midwife when she visits you postnatally;
- meet with a support service, such as: Patient Advice and Liaison Services (PALS), and in Scotland the Patient Advice and Support Service Scotland (PASS) or the Birth Afterthoughts (or similar) service, which offers women an opportunity to discuss their birth experience.

Some hospitals have established designated perinatal maternal mental health teams, to provide a rapid debriefing and birth trauma counselling service. Check your local hospital's website.

You may, however, want to make a formal complaint, in which case write to the hospital's Chief Executive and Director/Head of Midwifery, and keep a copy of your email or letter

Each country has its own complaints process so check your local advice services. AIMS, the Patients Association, and BirthRights all produce information leaflets and website advice.

When you are out of time for an investigation of your complaint

If you wish to make a formal complaint but feel unable to do so within the deadline of one year after the incident, and/or feel unable to meet the staff to discuss your care, you can write to the Chief Executive of the hospital. Copy the letter to the Director/Head of Midwifery along the following lines, <u>after</u> you have received a copy of your case notes:
"I wish to make a formal complaint about my care during the birth of my baby, I regret that I am unable to furnish the details at the moment as I am still traumatised from the experience, but I shall be putting in a full report in due course."

This means that you will then be able to address the details of the complaint without the pressure of fitting into the one-year time limit. The complaint, however, will not appear in the complaints statistics, but the hospital will still have to investigate. Do try to submit the details as soon as you can. The longer you leave it the more difficult it is to investigate your complaint, as HPs move on or forget specific events.

Some women, like Louisa, found the experience of birth so traumatic that she could not face addressing it for many years. Even after this lengthy period she felt her complaint made a significant difference to the midwives' behaviour.

"I knew I had a year from her birth in which to make a complaint, so I revisited the idea close to her first birthday. I looked at the complaints procedure and allowed myself to think about the birth again. I discovered that I was still badly affected by the memory, and thinking about what the complaints procedure involved I realised I would not only be forced to revisit the memory many times if I initiated it, but I might also be required to face the staff I was complaining about, possibly in the building where it had occurred ... Even after a year, I did not feel up to taking this on emotionally. ... After four years, I reached a point where the memories did not induce an overwhelming emotional state, and we decided to have another child. The pregnancy brought back a lot of it [emotional turmoil], *mostly in the form of my crying over how I had allowed my own understanding and instincts to be over-ruled. ... I was*

not classed as having had a traumatic birth by hospital staff. The birth plan I wrote for my second birth that detailed it all for the first time seemed to come as a shock to those who read it, including my husband, who had had no idea how I had felt after our daughter's birth – he was another who I wanted to protect from the effects of my memories, and had a lot of influence over how I was treated the second time round. I don't know if my birth plan had any real effect on how others might have been treated, but for me and my family in isolation I don't think an official complaint would have been anything like as effective."

If you decide to make a complaint, it will at least ensure that the hospital will no longer be able to claim that *no-one has complained before.*

Resolving your complaint

If you are dissatisfied with your hospital or Health Board's investigation of your complaint, you have the right to complain to the Ombudsman (see Resources, Organisations).

The Ombudsman, however, does not have jurisdiction over private obstetric units, and if you have cause to complain about private care there is little choice other than writing to the director of the unit, or the only other option is to take legal action. See the section on Private Care on page 112.

Taking legal action

In order to take legal action against any care provider, you need to be able to show that there has been negligent treatment in your care. You can take legal action up to three years after the incident, or after the moment you first realised that there was negligence.

It is important that before you take any action you make a formal application, in writing, for your case notes. In the meantime, write down your memories of what happened, and encourage anyone else who was present to record what they saw or heard.

Should you decide to consult a lawyer, after receiving a copy of your case notes, it is important that you engage one who has experience in medical negligence cases. AvMA is a charity which gives free advice and support to those affected by possible medical negligence (see Resources, Organisations). It maintains a list of lawyers with medical negligence experience. This ensures that the lawyers are up-to-date and actively involved with medical negligence cases. A general or family solicitor, however helpful and understanding, may have little or no experience in the complexity of medical negligence law.

Private care

If you received private care you can complain to the director of the relevant unit and, if you are dissatisfied with their response, you can complain to the Independent Sector Complaints Adjudication Service (ISCAS), although not all independent healthcare providers are members (see Resources, Organisations).

Transforming maternity care

Whatever decisions you make following your experiences of care, you may find yourself becoming involved in helping to transform maternity care in various ways. In recent years, each country in the UK has supported various multidisciplinary organisations that consists of women and HPs working together to improve care locally:

England – Maternity Voices groups;

Scotland – Maternity Services Liaison Committees, and Patient Advice and Support Service;

Northern Ireland – Patient and Client Council;

Wales – Maternity Service Liaison Committees, and Community Health Councils.

A serious patient safety incident (SPSI)

A serious patient safety incident would include, for example, a woman having a major haemorrhage which endangered her life or a failure to alert senior HPs to a baby whose condition was deteriorating. While rare, SPSIs do happen.

NHS staff in England, Wales and Northern Ireland are encouraged to report all SPSIs to the National Reporting and Learning System (NRLS), and, in Scotland, to Adverse Incidents Scotland (AIS).

The NRLS collects and analyses information on patient safety incidents in the NHS. It then makes recommendations to reduce the risk of patient safety incidents. Such incidents are categorised as *"any unintended or unexpected incident which could have harmed or did lead to harm for one or more patients being cared for by the NHS."* The NRLS does not investigate each report individually but they provide feedback to the health service from time to time, based on its analysis and findings from all reports as a whole.

If you have a complaint which you think amounts to an SPSI, you can write to the hospital, ask them for a copy of their policy on serious incidents, and ask if they have investigated and reported the incident. If you are not satisfied with their response, you may wish to consider alerting NRLS yourself (see Resources, Organisations). This is worth doing, as the CQC has noted that "[there is a] *failure to review and learn from adverse events in the maternity services in some hospitals*" (Care Quality Commission, 2020).

Am I Allowed: 4th Edition

Chapter 10
When Things Don't Go to Plan: Difficult Outcomes

Sometimes, however well prepared, positive, and well cared for a woman is, pregnancy, labour and birth, and/or the time after birth, don't go straightforwardly. This chapter discusses some of the unexpected and unwanted outcomes that can happen. While these are unlikely to happen to you, some women feel that should they unexpectedly face difficult outcomes, being informed is helpful.

Extremely premature babies

One of the most difficult decisions facing parents and professionals are those that relate to babies that are born extremely prematurely – before 26 weeks. Parents suddenly find themselves in a situation where the survival of their baby is in question. They will find themselves having to consider what the long term outcome might be and the potential suffering that treatments may involve. For very premature babies, health professionals may realise that treatment is unlikely to be the right thing to do; but parents may not yet be ready to let their baby go. It is a very difficult situation for everyone involved.

If treatment is proposed, the parents of a very premature baby have the right to consider the interventions and treatment that HPs consider necessary, and the HPs have a professional obligation to fully inform the parents about what they consider to be the best course of action, bearing in mind that the outcome may be uncertain.

Current practice in most neonatal units in the UK is to resuscitate a baby who has reached 26 weeks, when the brain is developed sufficiently for damage to be less likely, and to provide intensive care until the outlook is clearer, but practice does vary, and resuscitation can be attempted before that. As life-saving treatment can be invasive, and may cause suffering, it is difficult for the paediatricians to know at the time whether this approach will be of benefit to the baby or not (Nuffield Council on Bioethics 2006), so they will be most concerned to discuss the best course of action with the parents. Parents of premature babies who live will face many decisions and challenges for some time to come. There are a number of local and national organisations to help if this happens to you (see under Resources).

Miscarriage

A miscarriage is defined as the unintended loss of a baby before the 24th week of pregnancy. Miscarriage in early pregnancy is very common, occurring in around one in six (15%) pregnancies. Most happen between the 6th and 10th week of pregnancy. Doctors sometimes call this a spontaneous abortion. This can be very upsetting to women who have lost a baby through miscarriage because the word abortion is usually associated with the deliberate termination of a pregnancy.

In Britain, when a baby dies in pregnancy before 24 weeks, there is no legal obligation to issue a death certificate and the baby cannot be registered. Many parents find this deeply upsetting, but since 2006 many hospitals have made arrangements for giving *certificates of commemoration* following RCOG advice (RCOG 2005).

Unless parents specify otherwise, most babies under 24 weeks will be cremated by the hospital as there are no statutory obligations about what happens to the baby's body. A few hospitals hold a service before cremating the baby and many parents have been helped by supportive clergymen, celebrants or other spiritual guides who have conducted a special memorial service for them.

Alternatively, you can take your baby home with you and make your own arrangements.

If parents decide to arrange for their baby to be cremated or buried, they will need a copy of the statement from the hospital saying that the baby was less than 24 weeks and showed no sign of life.

It may be distressing to know, but babies born this early are so small there may not be enough ashes remaining to be scattered.

A small number, around 1 in 100, of women will repeatedly miscarry (Mayo Clinic, 2020) and sometimes it is not possible to work out why. If that happens, you can ask for tests to be done to try to find the cause. As miscarriage is common, and often unexplainable, doctors might be reluctant to carry out these tests before a woman has had three miscarriages, and often they are unable to establish the cause.

Even after recurrent miscarriages, many women will carry a baby to term. In fact, a woman who has had a miscarriage is more likely to have a successful pregnancy next time than another miscarriage (Tommy's 2020).

Some women with a threatened miscarriage choose to stay in bed hoping that this will maintain the pregnancy, but there is no scientific evidence to show that bed rest makes any difference to the chances of maintaining their pregnancy.

Many women who have suffered a miscarriage are very keen to have an early ultrasound when they become pregnant again, to check that all is well with their pregnancy. Anxious about losing the current baby, some women then have repeated ultrasound examinations for reassurance, but this can sometimes increase anxiety (see Chapter 6 for information about ultrasound).

Unfortunately, women who miscarry are not routinely provided with support and often feel very anxious and unsupported.

It is not routine for health visitors to visit parents who have suffered a miscarriage, but if you feel you need some support and advice you can contact your local health visitor and ask for a visit and/or contact one of the support organisation (see Resources, Organisations).

Stillbirth and neonatal death

A stillbirth is the birth of a baby after the 24th week of pregnancy who neither breathes, nor shows any other sign of life following his or her birth. Whatever the stage of pregnancy, if a baby shows any sign of life at birth, for example breathes or has a heartbeat, then the baby must be registered as a live birth and a death.

Over 760,000 babies were born in the UK in 2019 of whom around one in 250 babies died.

In recent years the needs of grieving parents following a stillbirth have been recognised, and many hospitals have made special arrangements to support them. A photograph of the baby is usually taken, and kept in the case notes until parents are ready to see it (NHS Health 2018a). Hand and foot prints can also be obtained and kept as memories.

Cold cots may also be offered, giving parents a little longer with their baby – cold cots can be an option for some parents to take home (Smith et al 2020).

It is important that parents are supported to grieve in their own way, and while in the past there was sometimes uncertainty about the best way to do this, there has been much improvement in training in this area and specialist midwives are often able to give excellent care. If parents are feeling pressured into making a decision quickly, they have the right to state that they are not ready and will decide after they have had time to reflect.

If a baby is stillborn, the midwife or doctor will issue a medical certificate of stillbirth that enables parents to register the stillbirth of their baby. This should be done within 24 days of the birth. In Northern Ireland it should be done within a year. If parents wish to have their baby cremated they will need a doctor's signature on the Stillbirth Certificate, as undertakers currently cannot accept a midwife's signature.

A doctor's duty of care following the death of a baby at birth

In March 2004, Judge Gage, of the Queen's Bench Division, ruled that a doctor caring for a mother whose baby has died has a duty of care to advise the mother about future pregnancies, give some explanation of the purpose of the post-mortem and explain what is involved (Powell v Boladz 1997). This ruling still stands.

The doctor also has a duty to explain whether or not any of the baby's organs will be retained.

If parents refuse to agree to a post-mortem, they can instead discuss with their doctor other tests that could be undertaken that may give some information about the cause of death.

Post-mortem (autopsy) examination

The purpose of a full post-mortem examination is to look for any medical condition that could have led to the death of the baby; it can also rule out any diseases or abnormalities which parents may have suspected or feared.

Post-mortems need to be done within 72 hours of a baby's death. If the baby's death occurred during, or shortly after, the birth it is important for the pathologist to examine the placenta as well. It is important that the post-mortem is done by a specialist neonatal pathologist, otherwise essential information may be missed.

Following a post-mortem the pathologist will write a preliminary report, which will be sent (within two weeks) to the Coroner, if she or he is involved, or to the doctor responsible for the baby's care. Parents are entitled to a copy of this report. Test results, however, can take up to six to 12 weeks to arrive if special tests are undertaken.

Parents have a right to accept or refuse a post-mortem (also called an autopsy examination) except in circumstances where the police believe it may be a suspicious death, in which case HPs have a duty to notify the

Coroner, who may then authorise a post-mortem without the parents' consent. Although making decisions immediately after losing a baby is difficult, some parents do exercise their right to refuse one.

If a post-mortem is carried out, then parents can inform the pathologist in writing that they reserve the right to have a second independent post-mortem performed if they disagree with the results, although there is no automatic right to a second post-mortem (Coroners Society of England and Wales, 2019).

Parents are entitled to see and hold their baby after the post-mortem has taken place, if that's what they wish. They can discuss this decision with a trusted professional who will dress the baby in their chosen clothes.

A Coroner's inquiry

If a baby is born dead, parents have no right to go to the Coroner, even if they think there was negligence. If the baby lived for a short a time, and poor care was thought to contribute to the death, a complaint can be made to the Coroner with a request for an inquiry. Those who wish to do this should first obtain a copy of the mother's and baby's case notes, and then consult AvMA (see Resources, Organisations).

Dealing with grief

Some parents feel that they are alone in their grief, miles away from their family and friends, and do not know who to turn to for help. SANDS (called Held in our Hearts in Lothian), Child Bereavement UK, the local Maternity Voices Partnership, or MSLC, CHC, or their local Citizen's Advice Bureau, may be able to help and put them in touch with local parents who have had a stillbirth or neonatal death. Parents can also ask their GP about local counselling services. Another option is to pay for individual counselling or psychotherapy. Counsellors and psychotherapists vary, as do their fees. It is important to find the right person, so asking around for recommendations from people who may know could be helpful.

Court ordered caesareans

In April 1996, Ms S, a thirty-year old veterinary nurse, registered with a new GP. She was 36 weeks pregnant and the GP diagnosed that she was suffering from pre-eclampsia and insisted that she be admitted to hospital immediately for induction of labour. She disagreed with his diagnosis and refused to be admitted. The GP contacted a social worker and an application was made to detain her under the Mental Health Act.

Ms S persisted in her refusal to have treatment and the staff then made an application for a Court Order to carry out an emergency caesarean. The Judge was told that this was a *"life and death situation and with only minutes to spare"*. This was untrue. No questions were asked about Ms S's competence, and she was not present in court. She was detained in a mental health unit and was not visited by a midwife during the three days prior to the caesarean surgery. Clearly, not a *life and death situation*.

Following the caesarean, Ms S challenged the judgement and appealed to the High Court. The Appeal Court ruled that the hospital's action was unlawful and she was awarded £40,000 damages.

The High Court was so concerned by this case that it issued guidelines to doctors, nurses, midwives and lawyers advising them on appropriate action should a similar situation ever arise again, and reminding them that a woman has the right to refuse treatment, and cannot be forced to undergo treatment unless it can be clearly demonstrated that the woman is not rational or lacks capacity. The judge commented: *"A mentally competent woman may decline treatment even where that might lead to death or serious harm to her or her baby."* (Ms S v St George's Hospital 1998).

While very rare, if you are concerned that you are being threatened with a Court Order to enforce treatment, it is very important that you ensure that you have access to a lawyer and someone to support you, such as Legal Action for Women, The Family Rights Group, AIMS or BirthRights (see Resources, Organisations).

Conversely, in the judgment in Montgomery v Lanarkshire Health Board [2015] UKSC 11, paragraph 87, where a woman argued that she would have chosen caesarean surgery if she had been fully informed of the risks in her individual case, the court concluded that, *"The doctor is therefore under a duty to take reasonable care to ensure that the patient is aware of any material risks involved in any recommended treatment, and of any reasonable alternative or variant treatments."*

Postnatal depression (PND) and Post Traumatic Stress Disorder (PTSD)

Even when all goes well, some women suffer from *baby blues*, which generally involves feeling tearful and upset a few days after the birth. For the majority this soon passes, but some women can develop postnatal depression or PTSD as a result of their experiences during the birth or for other reasons.

PTSD was not diagnosed in new mothers until the 1990s, although I and other lay activists were aware of this condition before it was given a name. It has become a more accepted diagnosis and, in some areas, PTSD and PND are recognised as different conditions and some have designated perinatal maternal mental health teams to support women. In some areas, however, women struggling with PTSD are still being misdiagnosed as having postnatal depression.

Women who need to be hospitalised for treatment, more commonly for PND and/or psychosis than PTSD, should, whenever possible, have their babies (if they are under a year old) with them.

The Mental Health (Care and Treatment) (Scotland) Act (2003) requires that all women admitted to inpatient psychiatric services have the opportunity to have their babies, if under one year, admitted with them. There are no similar legal requirements in England, Wales, or Northern Ireland. If you find that you are expected to be admitted without your baby you, and your family, can ask to talk to the senior doctor, point out the benefits of keeping mothers and babies together and ask why this is not being offered. You can also contact local or national support groups (see Resources, Organisations).

Many years ago, psychiatrist and AIMS member, Dr Desmond Bardon, developed the first Mother and Baby Unit in Hitchen, Hertfordshire, which was specifically designed to keep mothers and babies together while the mother received treatment for postnatal depression or postnatal psychosis. Many more of these specialist mother and baby units were developed, but during the 1990s almost all of these units were closed down, at a time when hospitals were trying to save money.

Recently, because of greater awareness of the importance of the mother baby relationship and the increasing numbers of women suffering from postnatal problems, these units have been established once again, in England, where there are 15, and in Scotland, where there are two. Currently, Northern Ireland and Wales have none.

Reporting suspected adverse drug reactions

Adverse drug reactions should be reported to the Medicines and Healthcare Products Regulatory Agency (MHRA) via the Yellow Card System (see Resources, Organisations). You can do this online if you wish (MHRA 2020) or download a form and send it to the MHRA via freepost (see Resources, Websites).

This includes any adverse reactions experienced by a mother during pregnancy, labour and postnatally, and for adverse reactions experienced by the baby, including adverse reactions to vaccinations.

"It is sometimes necessary for women to take medicines while pregnant. Some women may take medicines before they know they are pregnant. [...] it is important to collect reports of suspected adverse reactions experienced by the woman or child associated with medicines taken during pregnancy." (Medicines and Healthcare Products Regulatory Agency 2014).

Am I Allowed: 4th Edition

Thirty-five percent of systematic reviews of health care interventions changed, partially reported, or excluded adverse reactions in their registered protocols (Parsons 2018). This is why it is important for people to report an adverse effect themselves.

If you think that a medicine, vaccination, or other drug has caused an adverse side effect you can also report this to your GP, pharmacist, or whoever prescribed the drug, as well as the MHRA.

Last Words

Until relatively recently, it had been assumed that our current industrialised system of centralised and medicalised hospital birth is safe and the best way to organise maternity services. It is only relatively recently that an overwhelming body of good quality international research has been gathered and assimilated to show very clearly that continuity of midwifery care improves outcomes for all women and babies, no matter where a woman gives birth, and that improvements for healthy women and babies are increased if they birth at home or in small FMUs.

While official statements of all kinds accept implicitly or explicitly both that continuity of carer is ideal, and that that birth at home or in a midwifery unit is the best choice for many women, there are still major challenges ahead, persuading Governments to provide funding for these changes and supporting HPs to work in new ways.

The history of community based, caseloading midwifery care, and small FMUs is both heartening and dispiriting. Caseloading or continuity midwifery teams have been frequently initiated but have often failed due to overly large caseloads, lack of autonomy for midwives over their work patterns, and health service cutbacks when they are seen as desirable but not essential by trusts. Midwifery units have been established with much enthusiasm, and then closed down within a few years because of pressures elsewhere in the service and lack of referrals due to prejudice against them. Despite the evidence of better outcomes for birth in the community for healthy women, more large, centralised obstetric units are being created by the closure of smaller obstetric units. This is often in the face of local opposition, and despite the evidence that such care is not appropriate for the majority of fit and healthy women and babies.

Campaigning for change

Changing maternity service provision takes time, particularly in an organisation as centralised, and as under-resourced, and under threat of privatisation as the NHS (El-Gingihy 2018).

While the UK government has accepted that continuity of midwifery carer leads to better outcomes for mothers and babies and that out of hospital birth should be a realistic option for women, there are still major challenges ahead. Governments need to be persuaded to provide adequate funding for these changes to be initiated and sustained. Although continuity of midwifery carer will produce substantial savings in time, there needs to be initial funding and good leadership to support and encourage midwives and others to work in new ways.

Research from all over the world has unequivocally shown that women and babies have better outcomes, fewer interventions and are more satisfied with their care when they receive continuity of midwifery care from skilled midwives who are themselves well-resourced and have autonomy over their own work patterns.

For the necessary changes to maternity services to happen we need to identify and look to examples throughout the country of superb initiatives and achievements.

The provision of maternity care will only change when individual women and HPs keep pressing for change. Not only is your voice important, but it is also important to support those within the system who are trying to change it.

You can add your voice to those who are campaigning for change. When you are deciding where to give birth you can contact your hospital, Trust, Health Board or the Clinical Commissioning Group, and ask them what provision they have made for you to have continuity of carer with a case-load midwife, who will be responsible for caring for you throughout your pregnancy, birth, and postnatally.

If the claim is that such provision is more expensive, you can suggest that that may be true in the short term, but in the long-term there are enormous benefits for the health and wellbeing of mothers, babies and families, as well as cost benefits to the NHS. You can also consider contacting your local Maternity Voices Partnership group, MSLC, or other local or national support groups (see Resources, Organisations) and contact your local MP or MSP to ask them to take up the matter.

Whatever your experience of birth, do write and tell the Director/Head of Midwifery and the hospital Board or Trust Director about it. If your experience is good it will encourage the staff; if it is not so good they will have an opportunity to improve.

Whatever shape your pregnancy and birth journey takes, having a positive experience is very important, as the memories will remain with you for the rest of your life. It is your body, your baby, and you are entitled to the best possible care during this important time.

Am I Allowed: 4th Edition

Resources

Organisations

Action Against Medical Accidents (AvMA)
www.avma.org.uk

Association of Breastfeeding Mothers (ABM)
www.facebook.com/AssocBfMothers/

Association for Improvements in the Maternity Services (AIMS)
www.aims.org.uk

Birth Practice and Politics Forum
www.birthpracticeandpolitics.org

Birthrights
www.birthrights.org.uk

Breastfeeding Network (BfN)
www.breastfeedingnetwork.org.uk

Child Bereavement UK
www.childbereavementuk.org

Citizens Advice (formerly known as CAB – Citizens Advice Bureau)
www.citizensadvice.org.uk

Community Health Council (CHC) Wales
www.nhsdirect.wales.nhs.uk/localservices/communityhealthcouncils/

Family Rights Group
www.frg.org.uk/need-help-or-advice

Independent Midwives UK (IMUK)
www.independentmidwives.org.uk

Am I Allowed: 4th Edition

Independent Sector Complaints Adjudication Service (ISCAS)
www.idf.uk.net/content/documents/complaints/iscas-patient-guide-for-making-complaints%20(1).pdf

Information Commissioner
ico.org.uk/for-the-public/personal-information/

Lactation Consultant of Great Britain (IBCLC)
www.lcgb.org

La Leche League
www.laleche.org.uk

Legal Action for Women
legalactionforwomen.net/about/

Local Government Ombudsman
www.lgo.org.uk

MHRA – Medicines and Healthcare Products Regulatory Agency – Yellow Card Report
yellowcard.mhra.gov.uk

Maternity Action –Maternity Rights Advice Line (for employment rights)
maternityaction.org.uk/advice-line/

Maternity Voices Partnerships – England
nationalmaternityvoices.org.uk

Miscarriage Association
www.miscarriageassociation.org.uk

National Childbirth Trust
www.nct.org.uk

National Breastfeeding Helpline
www.facebook.com/nationalbreastfeedinghelpline

National Reporting and Learning System (Office of National Statistics) England and Wales
improvement.nhs.uk/resources/report-patient-safety-incident/

what every woman should know **before** she gives birth

National Reporting and Learning System (NRLS) Northern Ireland
www.health-ni.gov.uk/articles/reporting-adverse-incident

Positive Birth Movement
www.positivebirthmovement.org

Pregnancy and Parents Centre – Edinburgh
pregnancyandparents.org.uk

Private Midwives
privatemidwives.com

Refuge
www.refuge.org.uk

Stillbirth and Neonatal Death Society (SANDS)
www.sands.org.uk

UK Association for Milk Banking
www.ukamb.org

White Ribbon Alliance
www.whiteribbonalliance.org/wp-content/uploads/2017/11/Final_RMC_Charter.pdf

Women's Aid
www.womensaid.org.uk
www.nationaldahelpline.org.uk

Ombudsmen

Ombudsmen for health complaints

England
Parliamentary and Health Service Ombudsman
tel: 0345 015 4033
www.ombudsman.org.uk

Northern Ireland
Northern Ireland Public Services Ombudsman

Am I Allowed: 4th Edition

tel: 0800 34 34 24 or 02890 233821
nipso.org.uk/nipso/

Scotland
Scottish Public Services Ombudsman
tel: 0800 377 7330 or 0131 225 5300
www.spso.org.uk

Wales
Public Services Ombudsman for Wales
tel: 0300 790 0203
www.ombudsman-wales.org.uk

Ombudsmen for social services complaints

England
Local Government and Social Care Ombudsman
tel: 0300 061 0614
www.lgo.org.uk/contact-us

Scotland
Patient Advice and Support Service Scotland (PASS)
www.careinfoscotland.scot/topics/your-rights/patient-advice-and-support-service-pass/

Northern Ireland
Patient and Client Council Northern Ireland
www.patientclientcouncil.hscni.net

Websites and Links

Birth Practice and Politics Forum
www.birthpracticeandpolitics.org

Fear Free Childbirth
www.fearfreechildbirth.com/blog/cord-clamping-why-we-need-to-wait-for-white-with-amanda-burleigh/

Medicines and Healthcare Products Regulatory Agency (MRHA)
yellowcard.mhra.gov.uk

Public Health England (PHE) Screening
phescreening.blog.gov.uk/2017/08/24/midwives-are-you-discussing-residual-blood-spots-with-parents/

Postnatal check
www.nhs.uk/conditions/pregnancy-and-baby/newborn-physical-exam/

Ted Talk
www.youtube.com/watch?v=Cw53X98EvLQ

Vaccinations – routine vaccinations for babies and toddlers
www.nhs.uk/conditions/vaccinations/

WHICH?
www.which.co.uk/birth-choice

Maternity policies

England
National Maternity Review (2016). Better Births. Improving outcomes in maternity services in England. A 5-year forward view for maternity care, www.england.nhs.uk/publication/better-births-improving-outcomes-of-maternity-services-in-england-a-five-year-forward-view-for-maternity-care/

Northern Ireland
Northern Ireland Regulation and Quality Improvement Authority (2017). Review of strategy for maternity care in Northern Ireland 2012-2018, Department of Health, March 2017
www.health-ni.gov.uk/publications/strategy-maternity-care-northern-ireland-2012-2018

Scotland
Scottish Government (2017). The best start: maternity and neonatal care plan executive summary.

Am I Allowed: 4th Edition

www.gov.scot/publications/best-start-five-year-forward-plan-maternity-neonatal-care-scotland-9781786527646/

Wales
Welsh Government (2019). Maternity Care in Wales. A five year vision for the future (2019-2024).
gov.wales/sites/default/files/publications/2019-06/maternity-care-in-wales-a-five-year-vision-for-the-future-2019-2024.pdf

Books

There is a huge variety of birth books on the market. Many have been written by doctors or journalists who have little understanding of the issues in the maternity services, and many of these books seem designed to encourage you to unquestioningly accept whatever is on offer. There is a growing number of books written by expert lay people with a more questioning attitude, or by professionals who fully support the concept of informed choice. The following are some recommended books:

50 Human Studies in utero, conducted in Modern China indicate extreme risk for Prenatal Ultrasound – A New Bibliography by Jim West, (2015), Library of Congress Control Number 944054, ISBN 978-1-941719-03-9.

Birth in Focus by Becky Reed (2016), Pinter and Martin, ISBN 978-1-78066-235-02015.

Birthing Your Baby – the second stage of labour by Nadine Pilley Edwards (2019), Third Edition, Birth Practice and Politics Forum, Edinburgh, ISBN-10:1-9160606-1-7.

Birthing Your Placenta – The Third Stage of Labour by Nadine Edwards and Sara Wickham (2018), 4th Edition, Birthmoon Creations, Avebury and Edinburgh, ISBN-10:1999806441.

Breech Birth – what are my options? by Jane Evans J (2005), Association for Improvements in the Maternity Services, London, ISBN 10: 1874413177.

what every woman should know **before** she gives birth

Breech Birth Woman Wise by Maggie Banks (1998), Birth Spirit Publications, Hamilton, New Zealand, ISBN0-473-04991-0.

Group B Strep Explained by Sara Wickham (2019), 2nd edition, Birth Moon Creations, Avebury, ISBN 978-1999806422.

How to dismantle the NHS in 10 easy steps by Youssef El-Gingihy (2018), 2nd Edition, ISBN 978-1-78904-178-1.

Ina May's Guide to Childbirth by Ina May Gaskin (2008), Vermilion, 13579108642.

Inducing Labour – Making Informed Decisions by Sara Wickham (2018), 2nd Edition, Birthmoon Creations, ISBN-10: 9998064-.

Informed Choice in Maternity Care Ed. Mavis Kirkham (2004), Palgrave MacMillan, ISBN 0-333-99843-X.

Informed is Best: how to spot fake news about your pregnancy, birth and baby by Amy Brown (2019), Pinter and Martin, ISBN 978-1-78066-490-3.

Kangaroo Babies: A different way of mothering by Nathalie Charpak and Elfreda Powell, (2006), Souvenir Press, London, ISBN 9780285639331.

Optimal Care in Childbirth: The case for physiologic approach by Henci Goer and Amy Romano (2013), Pinter and Martin, London, ISBN 9781780661100.

Overdue, Birth, burnout and a blueprint for a better NHS by Amity Reed, Pinter and Martin (2020), ISBN 978-1-78066-410-1.

Revisiting Waterbirth – An Attitude to Care by Dianne Garland (2017), 2nd Edition, Palgrave, ISBN 978-1-137-60494-1.

Saying Goodbye to your baby: For parents who have had a late miscarriage, stillbirth or neonatal death by SANDS (2013), Stillbirth and Neonatal Death Charity.

The Positive Breastfeeding Book – Everything you need to feed your baby with confidence by Amy Brown (2018), Pinter and Martin, ISBN 978-1-78066-460-6.

Am I Allowed: 4th Edition

The Positive Birth Book Visual Birth Plan Cards by Milli Hill, Pinter and Martin, ISBN 9781780663142.

Vitamin K and the Newborn by Sara Wickham (2017), Birthmoon Creations, 2nd Edition, ISBN-10; 1999806409.

What's Right for Me? Making decisions in pregnancy and childbirth, by Sara Wickham (2018), Birthmoon Creations, 2nd edition, ISBN-10:1999806417.

Why Homebirth Matters by Natalie Meddings (2018), Pinter and Martin, ISBN 978-1-78066-555-9.

Why Induction Matters by Rachel Reed (2019), Pinter and Martin, London.

References

Alfirevic Z, Stampalija T and Medley N (2015). Doppler ultrasound of fetal blood vessels in normal pregnancies. Cochrane Database of Systematic Reviews. pubmed.ncbi.nlm.nih.gov/20687066/

Alfirevic Z, Devane D, Gyte GML, et al (2017). Continuous cardiotocography (CTG) as a form of electronic fetal monitoring (EFM) for fetal assessment during labour. Cochrane Database of Systematic Reviews 2017, Issue 2. Art. No: CD006066. doi: 10.1002/14651858.CD006066.pub3.

Allen J, Kildea S, Tracy MB et al (2019). The impact of caseload midwifery, compared with standard care, on women's perceptions of antenatal care quality: Survey results from the M@NGO randomized controlled trial for women of any risk, Birth. onlinelibrary.wiley.com/doi/abs/10.1111/birt.12436

Allmark P (2006). Choosing health and the inner citadel, J Med Ethics; 32: p3-6.

Ang ESBC Jr, Gluncic V, Duque A et al (2006). Prenatal exposure to ultrasound waves impacts neuronal migration in mice, Proceedings of the National Acadamy of Science of the United States 12903-12910.

Anim-Somuah M, Smyth RMD, Cyna AM and Cuthbert A (2018). Epidurals for pain relief in labour, Cochrane Database of Systematic Reviews, Cochrane Library. doi.org/10.1002/14651858.CD000331.pub4

Arnon S, Diamant C, Bauer S et al (2014). Maternal singing during kangaroo care led to autonomic stability in preterm infants and reduced maternal anxiety. Acta Paediatrica, John Wiley & Sons Ltd, first published online, 11 AUG 2014, doi: 10.1111/apa.12744.

Ashrafganjooei T, Naderi T, Eshrati B et al (2010). Accuracy of ultrasound, clinical and maternal estimates of birth weight in term women, Eastern Mediterranean Health Journal, Vol 16, No3, p313-317.

Beech BAL and Robinson J (1994). Ultrasound Unsound? Association for Improvements in the Maternity Services, London.

Beech BAL (2014). Ultrasound: an overused, under-researched technology, AIMS Occasional Paper, Association for Improvements in the Maternity Services, London.

Beech B A (2019). Informed consent for giving birth in hospital, Birth Practice and Politics. www.birthpracticeandpolitics.org/post/2019/05/29/informed-consent-for-giving-birth-in-hospital

Bello SO and Ekele BA (2012). On the safety of diagnostic ultrasound in pregnancy: Have we handled the available data correctly? Annals of African Medicine, Vol 11, No 1, p1-4.

Birthrights (2017). Consenting to treatment, Birthrights, London.

Birthrights (2017a). Unassisted birth, Birthrights, London.

Bohren MA, Hofmeyr GJ, Sakala C, et al (2017) Continuous support for women during childbirth. Cochrane Database of Systematic Reviews, Issue 7. Art. No.: CD003766. doi: 10.1002/14651858.CD003766.pub6.

Brocklehurst P, Hardy P, Hollowell J et al (2011). Perinatal and maternal outcomes by planned place of birth for healthy women with low risk pregnancies: The Birthplace in England national prospective cohort study' BMJ, Vol.343 (No.7840). d7400. ISSN 0959-535X.

Bronsteen R, Valice R, Lee W et al (2009). Effect of a low-lying placenta on delivery outcome, doi.org/10.1002/uog.6304: 27 January 2009.

Brown, A. (2016). Breastfeeding Uncovered: Who really decides how we feed our babies? Pinter & Martin www.pinterandmartin.com/breastfeeding-uncovered.html

Brown A (2018). The Positive Breastfeeding Book — Everything you need to feed your baby with confidence, Pinter and Martin, ISBN 978-1-78066-460-6.

Brownlee S, Chalkidou, Doust J et al (2017). Evidence for overuse of medical services around the world, The Lancet, Vol 390, p156-68.

Buckley SJ (2005). Epidurals: Risks and concerns for mother and baby, Dr Sarah Buckley. sarahbuckley.com/epidurals-risks-and-concerns-for-mother-and-baby/

Buckley SJ (2015). Hormonal Physiology of Childbearing: Evidence and Implications for Women, Babies, and Maternity Care. Washington, D.C.: Childbirth Connection Programs, National Partnership for Women & Families, January 2015.

Burleigh A (2012). Delaying the clampers, AIMS Journal, Vol 24, No4, p13, 14.

Burleigh A (2020). Wait for White. waitforwhite.com/about-amanda-burleigh/

Burns EE, Boulton MG, Cluett E et al (2012). Characteristics, Interventions, and outcomes of women who used a birthing pool: A prospective observational study, Birth, 39, p192-202, 3 Sept 2012.

Burns E, Feeley C, Venderlaan J et al (2020). Coronavirus COVID-19: Supporting healthy pregnant women to safely give birth, Oxford Brookes University, Oxford.

Camargo JCS, Varela V, Ferreira FM et al (2017). The waterbirth project: Sao Bernardo Hospital experience, Women and Birth, Vol 31, Issue 5, p325-e333.

Çankaya S and Şimşek B (2020. Effects of antenatal education on fear of birth, depression, anxiety, childbirth self-efficacy, and mode of delivery in primiparous pregnant women: A prospective randomized controlled study, Clinical Nursing Research, Sage Journals, April 2020. journals.sagepub.com/doi/10.1177/1054773820916984

Care Quality Commission (2018). 2017 survey of women's experiences of maternity care, Care Quality Commission, Maternity Services Survey, Statistical Release, Independent Data Analysis. January 2018.

Care Quality Commission (2020). Getting safer faster; key areas for improvement in maternity services. www.cqc.org.uk/publications/themed-work/getting-safer-faster-key-areas-improvement-maternity-services

Charpak N and Powell E (2006). Kangaroo Babies: A different way of mothering, Souvenir Press, London, ISBN 9780285639331.

Cheng YV, Shaffer BL, Nicolson JM and Caughey AB (2014). Second stage of labor and epidural use: A larger effect than previously suggested, Obstet Gynecol, 123(3) p527-35.

Cheyne H, Critchley A, Elders A et al (2015). Having a baby in Scotland 2015: listening to mothers, National Report, An Official Statistics publication for Scotland, Scottish Government.

Cluett ER, Burns E (2009). Immersion in water in labour and birth. Cochrane Database Syst Rev. 2009. doi:10.1002/14651858.CD000111.pub3. [PMC free article] [PubMed].

Cluett ER, Burns E Cuthbert A (2018). Immersion in water during labour and birth, Cochrane Database Syst Rev. 2018, Issue 5. Art.NO.:CD000111.doi:10.1002/14651858.CD000111.pub4.

Coroners' Society of England and Wales (2019). Chief Coroner Guidance 32 – Post-mortem examination, including 2nd Post-mortems, 23 Sept, 2019.

Cotzias CS, Paterson-Brown S and Fisk N (!999). Prospective risk of unexplained stillbirth in singleton pregnancies at term population: based analysis, British Medical Journal, Vol 319, p287-8.

Coxon K, Chisholm, A, Malouf R et al (2017). What influences birth place preferences, choices and decision-making amongst healthy women with straightforward pregnancies in the UK? A qualitative evidence synthesis using a 'best fit' framework approach, BMC Pregnancy and Childbirth, 17, Article number: 103.

Data Protection Act (2018). Legislation, Gov.uk, www.gov.uk/data-protection

Davies S (2011). Troubled Waters? AIMS Journal, Vol 23, No 4, p17-18.

Dawes GS. Foetal and Neonatal Physiology: A Comparative Study of the Changes at Birth. Chicago, IL: Yearbook Medical Publishers Inc., 1968.

De Benedictis S, Johnson C, Roberts J et al (2018). Quantitative insights into televised birth: a content analysis of One Born Every Minute, Critical Studies in Media Communication, 36:1, 1-17, doi: 10.1080/15295036.2018.1516046.

Devane D, Lalor JG, Daly S et al (2017). Comparing electronic monitoring of the baby's heartbeat on a woman's admission in labour using cardiotocography (CTG) with intermittent monitoring, Cochrane, Primary Review Group, Pregnancy and Childbirth Group.

Dixon L, Fletcher I, Tracy S et al (2009). Midwives care during the third stage of labour: an analysis of the New Zealand College of Midwives Midwifery Database 2004-2008. New Zealand College of Midwives Journal 41: 20-25.

Downe S, McCormick and Beech BL (2001). Labour interventions associated with normal birth, British Journal of Midwifery, Vol 9, No 10, p602-606.

Downe S, Gyte GM, Dahlen HG and Singata M (2013). Routine vaginal examinations for assessing progress of labour to improve outcomes for women and babies at term, Cochrane Database Syst Rev, Jul 15 (7). doi: 10.1002/14651858.pub2, CD010088.

Am I Allowed: 4th Edition

Downe S and Finlayson K (2016). Interventions in normal labour and birth, Survey Report March 2016, Royal College of Midwives.

Drandić and Leeuwen (2020). 'But a small price to pay' – Degradation of rights in childbirth during Covid-19, Oxford Human Rights Hub. ohrh.law.ox.ac.uk/but-a-small-price-to-pay-degradation-of-rights-in-childbirth-during-covid-19/

Edwards NP and Wickham S (2018). Birthing Your Placenta – the third stage of labour, 4th edition, Birthmoon Creations, Avebury and Edinburgh, ISBN -10: 1999806441.

Edwards NP (2019). Birthing your baby – the second stage of labour, Birth Practice and Politics Forum, Edinburgh, ISBN-10: 1-9160606-1-7.

Ewers H (2018). Maternity unit closures highlighted in new data, Royal College of Midwives, London.

Farrar D, Airey R, Law GR et al (2011). Measuring placental transfusion for term births: weighing babies with cord intact. BJOG. 118:70-75.

Finucane E, Murphy DJ, Biesty LM, et al (2020). Membrane sweeping for induction of labour, Cochrane, Pregnancy and Childbirth Group, 27 Feb 2020.

Fitzpatrick KE, Kurinczuk JJ, Bhattacharya S et al (2019). Planned mode of delivery after previous cesarean section and short-term maternal and perinatal outcomes: A population-based record linkage cohort study in Scotland, PLOS Medicine, doi: 10.1371/journal.pmed.1002913.

Frye A (1997). Understanding diagnostic tests in the childbearing year, Labrys Press, Oregon ISBN (paperback): 1.891145-50-9.

Gagnon JA and Sandall J (2007). Individual or group antenatal for childbirth or parenthood, or both, Cochrane Database of Systematic Reviews. www.cochranelibrary.com/cdsr/doi/10.1002/14651858.CD002869.pub2/full

Gallagher K, Martin J, Keller M et al (2014). European variation in decision-making and parental involvement during preterm birth, Arch Dis Child Fetal Neonatal Ed, 99(3); F246-9 doi: 10.1136/archdischild-2013-305191.

Garland D (2017). Revisiting Waterbirth: An attitude to care, 2nd edition, Palgrave, ISBN 978-1-137-60494-1.

Goer H (2015). Epidurals: Do they or don't they increase caesareans? Journal of Perinatal Education, Vol 24(4), p209-212.

Gov.uk (2020). Parental rights and responsibilities. www.gov.uk/parental-rights-responsibilities/who-has-parental-responsibility

Gupta JK, Sood A, Hofmeyr GJ et al (2017). Position in the second stage of labour for women without epidural anaesthesia, Cochrane Database of 'Systematic Reviews, doi: 10.1002/14651858.CD002006.pub4.

Harrison D Reszel J Bueno M et al (2020). Does breastfeeding reduce vaccination pain in babies aged 1 to 12 months? Cochrane Primary Review Group.

Henderson J, Burns EE, Regalia A et al (2014). Labouring women who used a birthing pool in obstetric units in Italy: prospective observational study, BMC Pregnancy and Childbirth 13, Article No 17.

Homer CSE, Leap N, Edwards N et al (2017). Midwifery continuity of carer in an area of high socio-economic disadvantage in London: A retrospective analysis of Albany Midwifery Practice outcomes using routine data (1997 – 2009), Midwifery 48, p1–10.

Hughes P, Turton P Hopper E et al (2002). Assessment of guidelines for good practice in psychosocial care of mothers after stillbirth: a cohort study, The Lancet 360(9327), p114-8. doi: 10.1016/s0140-6736(02)09410-2.

Hunter B, Henley J, Fenwick J et al (2018). Work, health and emotional lives of midwives in the United Kingdom: The UK WHELM study, School of Healthcare Sciences, Cardiff University.

Hutton EK, Reitsma A, Simioni J et al (2019). Perinatal or neonatal mortality among women who intend at the onset of labour to give birth at home compared to women of low obstetrical risk who intend to give birth in hospital: A systematic review and meta-analyses, The Lancet, Vol 14, p59-70.

Jukic AM, Baird DD, Weinberg CR et al (2013). Length of human pregnancy and contributors to its natural variation. Human Reproduction 2013 Aug 6, doi: 10.1093/humrep/det297.

Keulen JKJ, Bruinsma A, Kortekaas JC et al (2018). Timing induction of labour at 41 or 42 weeks? A closer look at time frames of comparison: a review. Midwifery, Vol 66, p111-118. www.sciencedirect.com/science/article/abs/pii/S0266613818302249?via%3Dihub

Khambalia AZ, Robers CL, Nguyen M et al (2013). Predicting date of birth and examining the best time to date a pregnancy, International Journal Gynecology Obstetrics, Vol 123, Issue 2, p105-109. doi: 10.1016/j.ijgo.2013.05.007. Epub 2013 Aug 6.

Kingsley C and McGlennan A (2017). The labour Epidural: Troubleshooting, Obstetric Anaesthesia, World Federation of Obstetric Anaesthesiologists, Tutorial 366.

Kirkham M (2019). Care, Birth Practice and Politics Forum, www.birthpracticeandpolitics.org/post/2019/09/04/care

Kordi M, Irani M, Tara F et al (2014). The diagnostic accuracy of purple line in prediction of labour progress in Omolbanin Hospital, Iran, Iran Red Crescent Medical Journals, Vol 16(11), e 16183, doi: 10.5812/ircmj.16183.

Kruske S, Young K, Jenkinson B and Catchlove A (2013). Maternity care providers' perceptions of women's autonomy and the law, BMC Pregnancy and Childbirth, 2013, 13:84 (2013), doi: 10.1186/1471-2393-13-84.

Lawrence A, Lewis L, Hofmeyr J et al (2013). Maternal positions and mobility during first stage labour, Cochrane Library, doi: 10.1002/14651858.CD003934.pub4.

Lindquist A, Kurinczuk JJ, Redshaw M et al (2014). Experiences, utilisation and outcomes of maternity care in England among women from different socio-economic groups: findings from the 2010 National Maternity Survey, British Journal of Obstetrics and Gynaecology.

obgyn.onlinelibrary.wiley.com/doi/10.1111/1471-0528.13059

Linton D (2017). Lacey Haynes, Experience: I had a freebirth, Life and Style, The Guardian, 28 April.

Liu Y, Liu Y, Huang Z et al (2014). A comparison of maternal and neonatal outcomes between water immersion during labor and conventional labor and delivery, BMC Pregnancy and Childbirth 2014, 14:160 doi: 10.1186/1471-2393-14-160.

Lukasse M, Rowe R, Townend J et al (2014). Immersion in water for pain relief and the risk of intrapartum transfer among low risk nulliparous women: secondary analysis of the Birthplace national prospective cohort study, BMC Pregnancy and Childbirth, 14:60(2014) doi: 10.1186/1471-2393-14-60.

Mayo Clinic (2020). Getting Pregnant. Pregnancy after miscarriage: what you need to know. www.mayoclinic.org/healthy-lifestyle/getting-pregnant/in-depth/pregnancy-after-miscarriage/art-20044134

MBRRACE-UK (2019). Saving lives, improving mothers' care, Mothers and babies: reducing risk through audits and confidential enquiries throughout the UK, National Perinatal Epidemiology Unit, Oxford.

McClintic AM, King BH, Webb SJ et al (2013). Mice exposed to diagnostic Eugenius ultrasound in utero are less social and more active in social situations relative to controls, Autism Research, vol 7 (3), p295-304.

Medical Defence Union (1974). Consent to Treatment, Medical Defence Union, London.

MHRA (2020). Yellow Card, Yellow Card Scheme, Medicines and Healthcare Products Regulatory Agency. yellowcard.mhra.gov.uk/

Middleton P, Shepherd E and Morris J et al (2018). Induction of labour at or beyond 37 weeks gestation, Cochrane Systematic Review – Intervention, July 2020.

Miller S, Abalos E, Chamillard M et al (2016). Beyond too little, too late and too much, too soon: a pathway towards evidence-based, respectful maternity care worldwide. Lancet 388(10056):2176-2192. doi: 10.1016/S0140-6736(16)31472-6.

Moore ER, Bergman N, Anderson GC et al (2016). Early skin-to-skin contact for mothers and their healthy newborn infants. Cochrane Database of Systematic Reviews 2016, Issue 11. Art. No.: CD003519. doi: 10.1002/14651858.CD003519.pub4.

Ms S v St George's Hospital (1998). Trust Guilty of Abuse of Power, St George's Hospital, Tooting, AIMS Journal Vol 10, No2, Summer 1998, p14-15.

Murphy Lawless (1998). Reading birth and death: a history of obstetric thinking, Cork University Press, ISBN 978-1859181768.

National Maternity and Perinatal Audit (2019). Organisational Report, 2019. maternityaudit.org.uk/FilesUploaded/NMPA%20organisational%20report%202019.pdf

National Maternity Review (2016). Better Births: Improving outcomes of Maternity Services in England, A five year forward view of maternity care.

www.england.nhs.uk/wp-content/uploads/2016/02/national-maternity-review-report.pdf

Nelson K, Sartwell T and Rouse D (2016). Electronic fetal monitoring, cerebral palsy, and caesarean section: assumptions versus evidence. BMJ 2016; 355:i6405 doi: 10.1136/bmj i6405.

NHS (2017). Common health questions, Do I have the right to refuse treatment? NHS Health A-Z.

NHS England (2017). A-EQUIP a model of clinical midwifery supervision, NHS England, p17.

NHS Digital (2019). NHS Maternity Statistics 2018-19, Summary Report, published October 2019.

NHS Digital (2020). Maternity Services Monthly Statistics, 1–31 March 2020, Experimental Statistics., published 25 June 2020.

NHS Health A-Z (2018). Healthy weight: BMI healthy weight calculator.

NHS Health A-Z (2018a). What happens if your unborn baby dies, NHS Health A-Z www.nhs.uk/conditions/stillbirth/what-happens/

NHS Health A-Z (2020). Your antenatal appointments, your pregnancy and baby guide, NHS A-Z.

NICE National Institute for Health and Care Excellence (2017). Intrapartum care for healthy women and babies, Clinical guideline CG 190, February, 1.1.2.

NICE National Institute for Health and Care Excellence (2019). Antenatal Care for uncomplicated pregnancies.

NICE National Institute for Health and Care Excellence (2019). Intrapartum care for women with existing medical conditions or obstetric complications and their babies, NICE guideline NG121.

NMC (2018). The Code, Professional standards of practice and behaviour for nurses and midwives, Nursing and Midwifery Council, London.

Northern Ireland Statistics and Research Agency (2017). www.nisra.gov.uk/publications/registrar-general-annual-report-2016-birthsobgyn.onlinelibrary.wiley.com/doi/10.1111/1471-0528.13059

NPMA (2017). National Maternity and Perinatal Audit, Clinical Report 2017, NMPA Project Team, RCOG London.

Nuffield Council on Bioethics (2006). Critical care decisions in fetal and neonatal medicine: ethical issues, Nuffield Council on Bioethics, ISBN 1 904383 14 5.

Odent M (2017). Home birth versus hospital birth: The bacteriological perspective, Midwifery Today, Vol 120, p16-18.

ONS (2019). Office of National Statistics, Annual Live Births England and Wales.

Parsons R, Golder S and Watt I (2018). More than one-third of systematic reviews did not report adverse events outcome. Journal of Clinical Epidemiology, Vol 108, p95-101.

Phin N (2017). Press Release, Alert after Legionnaires' disease case in baby, Public Health England.

Positive Birth Movement (2018). Campaigns, 40% of UK babies may not be getting Optimal Cord Clamping. www.positivebirthmovement.org/about/our-campaigns/

Powell S (2013). Holy meconium: a potted history, Essentially MIDIRS, Vol 4, No 9, p18-23.

Powell v Boladz (1997). 39 BMLR 35 distinguished, High Court, London BLD 2903041387; [2004] EWHC 644 (QB).

Prusova K, Churcher L, Tyler A et al (2014). Royal College of Obstetricians and Gynaecologists guidelines: How evidence-based are they? Journal of Obstetrics and Gynaecology, Nov 2014, 34(8), pp706-711. doi:10.3109/01443615.2014.920794.

Public Health Scotland (2020). Births in Scottish hospitals, year ending 31 March 2020. beta.isdscotland.org/find-publications-and-data/population-health/births-and-maternity/births-in-scottish-hospitals/Rance S, McCourt, Rayment J et al (2013). Women's safety alerts in maternity care: is speaking up enough? British Medical Journal, Vol 22, Issue 4.

RCOG (2005). Disposal following pregnancy loss before 24 weeks gestation, Good Practice Guide, No.5.

RCOG (2013). RCOG release: Pregnant women should be assessed for a small for gestational age fetus to identify those at high risk, Royal College of Obstetricians and Gynaecologists, 22 March.

RCOG (2015a). Birth after previous caesarean birth, Green Top Guideline No. 45. Royal College of Obstetricians and Gynaecologists, 1 October.

RCOG (2015b). Ultrasound from conception to 10+0 weeks' gestation, Scientific Impact Paper No.49, Royal College of Obstetricians and Gynaecologists, March 2015.

Reed R (2015). The curse of meconium stained liquor, Midwife Thinking. 14 January.

Reed R (2019). Cord blood collection: confessions of a vampire-midwife, Midwife Thinking. midwifethinking.com/2015/09/16/cord-blood-collection-confessions-of-a-vampire-midwife/

Roberts J (2020). A quarter of mothers' birth decisions were not respected, Mumsnet. www.mumsnet.com/news/quarter-of-mothers-birth-decisions-not-respected

Ross-Davie (2017). Evidence relating to place of maternity care, including place of birth, Scottish Government review. blogs.gov.scot/child-maternal-health/wp-content/uploads/sites/14/2019/03/Place-of-birth-evidence.pdf

Rowe RE, Kurinczuk J, Locock L et al (2012). Women's experience of transfer from midwifery unit to hospital obstetric unit during labour: a qualitative interview study, BMC Pregnancy and Childbirth, **12**, 129 (2012). bmcpregnancychildbirth.biomedcentral.com/articles/10.1186/1471-2393-12-129

Rowe RE, Townend J, Brocklehurst P et al (2013). Duration and urgency of transfer in births planned at home and in freestanding midwifery units in England: secondary analysis of the Birthplace national prospective cohort study, BMC Pregnancy and Childbirth, 13:224 doi: 10.1186/1471-2393-13-224.

Rowe R, Knight M, Brocklehurst P and Hollowell (2015). Maternal and perinatal outcomes in women planning vaginal birth after caesarean (VBAC) at home in England: secondary analysis of the Birthplace national prospective cohort study, BJOG, 2015; 123(7): 1123-32.

RPCPH (2020). BAMP- Covid-19: Frequently asked questions within neonatal services, Royal College of Paediatrics and Child Health, November 2020. www.rcpch.ac.uk/resources/bapm-covid-19-frequently-asked-questions-within-neonatal-services

Rydahl E, Declercq E, Juhl et al (2021). Routine induction in late-term pregnancies: follow-up of a Danish induction of labour paradigm, British Medical Journal Open, Vol 9 Issue 12, bmjopen.bmj.com/content/9/12/e032815

Saari-Kemppainen A, Karjalainen O, Ylöstalo P et al (1990). Ultrasound screening and prenatal mortality; controlled trial of systematic one-stage screening in pregnancy, The Lancet, Vol 339; p387-391.

Sandall J, Soltani H, Gates S et al (2016). Midwife-led continuity models of care versus other models of care for women during pregnancy, birth and early parenting, Cochrane Pregnancy and Childbirth Group, The Cochrane Library, 28 April. doi: 10.1002/14651858.CD004667.pub5.

Sandall J, Tribe RM, Mola G, Visser GHA et al (2018). Short-term and long-term effects of caesarean section on the health of women and children, The Lancet, Series – Optimising caesarean section use, Vol 392, Issue 10155, p1349-1347.

Sartwelle TP and Johnson JC (2014). Cerebral Palsy Litigation: Change course or abandon ship, Journal of Child Neurology, Vol 30:7, p828-841.

Sehgal A, Nitzan I, Jayawickreme N and Menaham S (2020). Impact of skin-to-skin parent-infant care on preterm circulatory physiology, Journal of Pediatrics, Vol 222, p91-97. www.jpeds.com/article/S0022-3476(20)303954/fulltext

Seijmonsbergen-Schermers, A, Scherjon S and de Jonge A (2019). Induction of labour should be offered to all women at term AGAINST: Induction of labour should not be offered to all women at term first: do no harm, BJOG Am International Journal of Obstetrics and Gynaecology.

Shallow H (2019). Is induction of labour morally justified? Birth Practice and Politics Forum. www.birthpracticeandpolitics.org/post/2019/03/25/is-induction-of-labour-morally-justifiable

Shepherd A, Cheyne H, Kennedy S et al (2010) The purple line as a measure of labour progress: a longitudinal study, BMC Pregnancy and Childbirth, 16 September.

Singata M, Tranmer J, Gyte GML (2013). Eating and Drinking in Labour, Cochrane Primary Review Group, 23 August.

Small K A, Sidebotham M, Fenwick J et al (2020). Intrapartum cardiotocograph monitoring and perinatal outcomes for women at risk: Literature review, Women and Birth.

www.sciencedirect.com/science/article/pii/S187151921930825X?via%3Dihub

Smith P, Vasileiou K and Jordan A (2020). Healthcare professionals' perceptions and experiences of using a cold cot following the loss of a baby: a qualitative study in maternity and neonatal units in the UK, BMC Pregnancy and Childbirth, 20, p175, doi: 10.1186/s12884-020-02865-4.

Stapleton H (2004). Is there a difference between a free gift and a planned purchase? The use of Evidence Based leaflets in Maternity Care. Chapter 5, p111, in Kirkham, Mavis (ed) Informed Choice in Maternity Care, Palgrave MacMillan.

Stewart D Ed. (1998). The Five Standards of Safe Childbearing, Marble Hill, MO: NAPSAC, P71.

Stuebe A (2020). Should infants be separated from mothers with Covid-19? First, do no harm. Breastfeeding Medicine. 15(5), p351-352. doi: 10.1089/bfm.2020.29153.ams.

Suman RPN, Udani R and Nanavati R (2008). Kangaroo mother care for low birth weight infants: A randomized controlled trial, Indian Pediatrics, 45(1), p17-23.

Tarantal AF, O'Brien WD and Hendricks AG (1993). Evaluation of the bioeffects of prenatal ultrasound exposure in the Cynomolgus Macacque (Macaca fascicularis): III Developmental and Mematologic Studies, Teratology, 1993, Vol 47, issue2, p159-170.

Teijlingen E et al. (2003) Maternity satisfaction studies and their limitations: 'What is, must still be best', Birth, Vol 30, Issue 2, p75-82.

Ternovszky v Hungary (2010) European Court of Human Rights, Second Section, Case of Ternovszky v. Hungary, Application No: 67545/09.

Tommy's (2020). Miscarriage Statistics. www.tommys.org/our-organisation/charity-research/pregnancy-statistics/miscarriage#recurrent

Ulfsdottir H, Saltvedt S and Georgsson S (2017). Waterbirth in Sweden – a comparative study, Acta Obstetricia et Gynecology Scandanavica, Vol 97, Issue 3, p341-348.

UN Report (2019). A human rights-based approach to mistreatment and violence against women in reproductive health services with a focus on childbirth and obstetric violence, United Nations General Assembly. undocs.org/A/74/137

UNICEF (2020). Minimising supplementation in the early days after birth, Education refresher pack during the coronavirus outbreak: Sheet 5, UNICEF. www.unicef.org.uk/babyfriendly/wp-content/uploads/sites/2/2020/05/Education-refresher-pack-sheet-5-minimising-supplementation-use-in-the-early-days-after-birth.pdf

Urashima M, Mezawa H, Okuyama M, et al (2019). Primary prevention of cow's milk sensitization and food allergy by avoiding supplementation with cow's milk formula at birth, JAMA Paediatr, published online 2019 Oct 21;173(12):1137-1145. jamanetwork.com/journals/jamapediatrics/fullarticle/2753281

Welsh Assembly Government (2011). A Strategic Vision for Maternity Services in Wales.p8. ISBN 978 0 7504 6627 1, Crown Copyright 2011.

Welsh Government (2019). Maternity and birth statistics: 2019. gov.wales/maternity-and-birth-statistics-2019

West J (2015). 50 human studies in utero, conducted in modern China indicate extreme risk for prenatal ultrasound. A new bibliography commentary, Library of Congress Control Number 2015944054. ISBN 978-1-941719-03-8.

West J (2017). Townsend Letter – The Examiner of Alternative Medicine. www.townsendletter.com/April2017/ultrasound0417.html

WHICH? (2019) Where to give birth. www.which.co.uk/birth-choice

WHO (1996). Safe Motherhood, Care in normal birth: a practical guide, Report of a technical working group, WHO/FRH/MSM/96.24.

WHO (2015a). WHO Statement on caesarean section rates, World Health Organization, WHO/RHR/15.02.

WHO (2015b). Caesarean sections should only be performed when medically necessary, WHO News release, World Health Organization, 10 April, Geneva.

WHO (2018). WHO recommendations: non-clinical interventions to reduce unnecessary caesarean sections, World Health Organization, ISBN: 978-92-4-155033-8.

WHO (2018a). WHO recommendations: induction of labour at or beyond term World Health Organisation, ISBN 978 92-4-155041-3.

WHO (2018b). WHO recommendation on skin-to-skin contact during the first hour after birth, World Health Organisation Reproductive Health Library, Geneva.

WHO (2020). Breastfeeding and Covid-19, Scientific Brief Geneva: World Health Organization, June 2020.

Wickham S (2019). Group B Strep Explained, Birthmoon Creations, Avebury, Wilts, ISBN-10:1999806425.

Winters P (2006). Holding up a mirror: the impact of user involvement, AIMS Journal, Vol 18, No3, 2006, p13.

Wyllie J, Ainsworth S and Tinnion R (2015). Guidelines: Resuscitation and support of transition of babies at birth, Resuscitation Council UK.

Zanetti-Dallenbach R, Lapaire O, Maertens A et al (2006). Water birth: is the water an additional reservoir for group B streptococcus? Archives of Gynecology and Obstetrics, Vol 273, Issue 4, p236-238.